Springer Series on Social Work

Albert R. Roberts, PhD, Series Editor

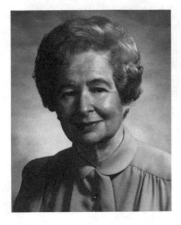

Risha W. Levinson, DSW, professor emerita, at the Adelphi University School of Social Work in Garden City, New York, holds a doctorate in social welfare from the Columbia University School of Social Work, and a master's degree in social service administration from the University of Chicago.

Dr. Levinson coauthored a book on *Accessing Human Services: International Perspectives* (Sage) in 1984 with Karen S. Haynes, PhD. In 1988, Dr. Levinson authored a textbook on *Information and Referral Networks: Doorways to Human Services* published by Springer.

Based on a federal grant that Dr. Levinson received from the U.S. Administration on Aging in 1984, she was the director of this library-based I&R training program, known as *Senior Connections*, which involved students and older volunteers. In 1995, this program was transferred from Adelphi to the Nassau Library System.

Dr. Levinson received the "Distinguished Service Award" from the Alliance of Information and Referral Services (AIRS) in 1990 for her contribution to the field of Information and Referral services and the AIRS organization. In 1991 Dr. Levinson was awarded an 18-month research grant in gerontology studies from the Gray Panthers to analyze intergenerational programs conducted jointly with older volunteers and interdisciplinary students in I&R internships. In 1992 Dr. Levinson was the recipient of the "Social Worker of the Year Award" as elected by the New York State Association of Social Workers.

Dr. Levinson has delivered many papers at conferences, conducted seminars and workshops on Information and Referral, and authored numerous articles and chapters in books related to practice issues and policy implications of I&R.

New Routes to Human Services

Information and Referral

Risha W. Levinson, DSW

 Springer Publishing Company

Springer Publishing Company, Inc.
536 Broadway
New York, NY 10012-3955

Acquisitions Editor: Sheri W. Sussman
Production Editor: Sara Yoo
Cover design by Susan Hauley

00 01 02 03 04 / 5 4 3 2 1

Library of Congress Cataloging-in-Publication Data

Levinson, Risha W.
    New routes to human services : information and referral / Risha W. Levinson.
        p. cm. — (Springer series on social work)
    Rev. ed. of: Information and referral networks. c1988.
    Includes bibliographical references and index.
    ISBN 0-8261-2393-7
    1. Human services—United States—Information services.   2. Social service—United States—Information services.   3. Public welfare—United States—Information services.
I. Levinson, Risha W. Information and referral networks.   II. Title.   III. Springer series on social work (Unnumbered)

HV29.82.U6 L49 2002
361.3'068—dc21   2001057552

Printed in Canada by Tri-Graphic Printing (Ottawa) Limited.

Contents

List of Tables and Figures

Acronyms

AARP	American Association of Retired Persons
AIRS	Alliance of Information and Referral Systems, Inc.
AoA	Administration on Aging
ARC	American Red Cross
AT&T	American Telephone and Telegraph Co., Inc.
CAB	Citizens Advice Bureaus
CIRS	Certified Information Referral Specialist
COS	Charity Organization Societies
CRS	Community Resource Specialist
DSS	Decision Support System
FCC	Federal Communications Commission
FIC	Federal Information Center
FSC	Family Support Centers
HCFA	Health Care Finance Administration
I&R	Information and Referral
IP	Internet Protocol
IT	Information Technology
LAN	Local Area Network
MIS	Management Information System
NACAB	National Association of Citizens Advice Bureaus
NASUA	National Association of State Units on Aging
OAA	Older Americans Act
PC	Personal Computer
SSA	Social Security Administration
TIP	The Information Place
UWA	United Way of America
UWASIS	United Way of America Services Identification System
VA	Veterans Administration
VICs	Veterans Information Centers
WWW	World Wide Web

Preface

This revised edition of the 1988 book on *Information and Referral Networks: Doorways to Human Services* has been designed to present an updated report on the continuous and dramatic expansion of Information and Referral (I&R) services that has occurred since its early beginnings in the 1960s. The current revised edition recognizes the enormous impact of information technology that has literally opened up new routes to the human services, thereby providing unprecedented opportunities for facilitating access to the complex systems of health and social services, jointly referred to as the human services.

Therefore, this updated edition bears the revised title of *New Routes to Human Services: Information and Referral* in recognition of the technological revolution, in addition to the social changes, demographic shifts, political realities, and new organizational patterns that have impacted on the nature and delivery of human services. Concurrently, the dramatic developments in information technology, particularly during the 1990s, have revolutionized the capabilities of providing I&R services at all levels of operations ranging from local communities to worldwide global levels. Consequently, the expansion of computerization within the human services presents opportunities to integrate social goals with technological developments that were almost unimaginable as recent as a decade ago.

The goal of this volume is to present a state-of-the-art report on Information and Referral that reflects the capabilities of information technology which have created new routes and new linkages to human services in response to the universal human need for information and helping services. In effect, this book represents a current comprehensive report that covers the 40-year development of I&R, beginning with the decade of the 1960s and expanding through 4 decades of dramatic growth of I&R services through the year 2000 with the new and dynamic applications of information technology.

The book is divided into four parts: Part I consists of three chapters that serve as background to the evolving and expanding fields of I&R and information technology. Chapter 1 defines the need and response of I&R to the complex world of human services. A schematic model of I&R (chap. 1, Figure 1.1) indicates that I&R responds to the universal, personal, and crisis-disaster needs of society with new routes to human services given the application of information technology. For purposes of background data, the subsequent two chapters provide an historical overview of the development and expansion of the fields of I&R (chap. 2) and information technology (chap. 3).

Part II consists of three chapters that present the basics of I&R operations in relation to service delivery, organizational variations, and the significant gains in professionalization through the certification of I&R specialists and organizational accreditation. Chapter 4 describes the components and the process of I&R service delivery with recognition of the emergence of an official tested taxonomy and the means for universal access to services through the utilization of the free, nationally approved 211 telephone number. Chapter 5 describes the variations and diversities of organized I&R services that have responded to the impact of the new technology in creating shared databases, organizational alliances, and service networks. In recognition of the current and anticipated expansion of the older population, chapter 6 describes new challenges for I&R services in light of the current and projected needs of a rapidly exploding aging population.

Part III relates directly to the practical tasks of instituting I&R services with the benefits of computerization and telecommunications. Chapter 7 suggests various I&R systems models that have the capacity to systematically apply information technology that has the capability to facilitate new routes for access to human resources. Chapter 8 focuses on the critical need for staffing and training of I&R personnel to provide essential "high touch" in service delivery plus the benefits of "high tech" in I&R service operations.

Part IV concludes with chapter 9, an Epilogue, which discusses trends, issues, constraints, and projections in providing new routes to human services, given the combined capabilities of I&R services and technological applications.

To meet the apparent need for a basic reader on I&R, this text combines both conceptual aspects and empirical reports on I&R developments. Since all human service helpers seek to facilitate access to existing services, this book suggests guidelines to services providers, to board members, and to social planners who are engaged in I&R provision and related human services. The content of the text is directed to professionals, paraprofessionals, and volunteers who are involved in I&R service delivery. For faculty and students in core curricula that deal with health and human services, this volume can serve as an informational resource and as an operational guide for class instruction, field internships, and social research. Since all persons are, at one time or another, users or potential consumers of I&R services, the interested reader may find the contents of this book useful to become a better informed citizen and to advocate for improved human services.

Acknowledgments

I t was my good fortune to have been one of the founders of the Alliance of Information and Referral Systems in the late 1960s and to continue as an active participant in the dynamic expansion of Information and Referral services. I am deeply indebted to my esteemed teacher and mentor, Alfred J. Kahn, professor emeritus of Social Policy, who first introduced me to the implications and challenges of organized access systems during my doctoral studies at the Columbia University School of Social Work. I also acknowledge the intellectual contribution of Nicholas Long, psychologist and researcher at Interstudy Associates, who first ventured to conceptualize I&R theory and practice in his research reports and bibliographical compilations on Information and Referral during the early 1970s.

I was privileged to share the enthusiasm of dedicated colleagues in the creation of AIRS under the energetic leadership of Corazon Estava Doyle, the first volunteer executive director of AIRS. I treasure the memory of meetings with Corazon in coffee shops at the Pennsylvania Railroad Station to jointly plan the agenda of the next year's annual meeting, which Corazon artfully outlined on paper napkins.

I am pleased to acknowledge the valuable contribution of Laura Zimmerman, director, Computer and Information Technology Unit, director, Human Services Smart Agency, at the School of Social Work, University of North Carolina at Chapel Hill, who authored chapter 7 on "Automating I&R: Some Nuts/Some Bolts." The content of this chapter reflects her rich experience as an educator, administrator, and researcher in I&R program development and systems design.

I gratefully acknowledge the contribution of Peter Liebscher, dean of the School of Library and Information Science at Catholic University in Washington, DC. Dean Liebscher and I conducted an interdisciplinary national survey on the complementarity of Social Work and Library Science in the delivery of I&R services (discussed in chap. 5). Dean Liebscher also submitted an early draft of chapter 3 on the history of information technology and I&R.

The many friends and associates whom I have met over the years and from whom I have learned so much are regrettably too numerous to list. However, I would like to mention some of the individual informants who have graciously shared their knowledge and experiences with me in the field of I&R. I would like to thank Ellen Evans from the United Way of America for her responses to my requests for information. To my colleagues at the Administration on Aging, both at NASUA and at the I&R Support Center, I thank Greg Case, Bernice Hutchinson, and Theresa Lambert for their helpfulness in providing me with information on the ever-expanding role of I&R/A services that continue to evolve and expand in the field of aging.

To my many friends and colleagues at AIRS, I owe a special note of appreciation for their challenges and accomplishments. I reserve a special commendation to Dick Manikowski for his thoughtful contribution to the literature of I&R, as editor of the AIRS Journal and compiler of bibliographical materials related to I&R. Manikowski has also made a valuable contribution in his "User Friendly" articles in the AIRS Newsletters on aspects of technology of I&R. I am also very appreciative of Georgia Sales' contribution as the founder and organizer of the AIRS/INFO LINE Taxonomy, a universal classification system of human services. Sales has also contributed thoughtful and challenging articles on the politics and policies of I&R in the AIRS Journal.

For the helpful compilation of the Chronology of AIRS that was published to honor the 25th Anniversary of AIRS in 1998, I thank Gil Evans, Warren Nance, and Hazel Smith. For coediting an early overview of international perspectives on I&R in our 1985 book on *Accessing Human Services: International Perspectives*, I convey my appreciation to my academic colleague, Karen S. Haynes, president of the University of Houston-Victoria, Texas.

I appreciate the Lifetime Honorary Membership Award which I received from the New York State Alliance of Information and Referral Services (NYSAIRS) in 1995, and have been very impressed with the creativity of the NYSAIRS Committee under the able presidency of Leta Weintraub.

My special recognition and thanks to Susan Sarnoff (currently assistant professor in the department of Social Work at Ohio University in Athens) for her accomplishments in the Senior Connections program as assistant administrator, research director, and student supervisor from 1989–1994. For the effective operation of Senior Connections during the first decade of operation (1985–1995), I gratefully acknowledge the professional contribution of three dynamic "retired" social workers–Edith Bigman, Anita Graber, and Gertrude Mayo.

Many thanks to the helpful reference librarians at the Adelphi University Swirbul Library and at the Garden City Public Library, with special mention of Martin Bowe of the reference staff who is also the coordinator for the Senior Connections program at the Garden City Public Library. For the continued operation and expansion of the I&R Senior Connections program at the Nassau County Library System since 1995, I acknowledge with appreciation the efforts of Dorothy Puryear, MLS (Manager, Special Library Services) and Francine Siegel, CSW (Project Director, Senior Connections).

I am pleased to add a special note of appreciation to my British friend, Sheila Bellamy, who hosted my site visits to Citizens Advice Bureaus during my two university sabbaticals in Great Britain in 1981 and 1989. I also thank Sheila for continuing to keep me informed on the NACAB program.

I convey special thanks to Tony W. R. Kosturi, a talented senior student in the Honors College at Adelphi University, who thoughtfully assisted me in the application of computer skills and in the organization and production of this text.

I am grateful to Albert R. Roberts, Social Work Editor for Springer Publishing, for his wise counsel and guidance in initially recognizing the need for a text on Information and Referral, which led me to write the first edition of this book in 1988. I especially appreciate his conviction on the importance of an updated report on I&R, particularly in light of the dramatic advances in information technology and the professionalization of I&R that have led to new routes to human services.

I express deep appreciation to my personal family members, including my four adult children and their spouses, and to my six *cheering grandchildren*, all of whom have lavished me with their enthusiasm in my dedication to the field of I&R. To Gerald, my husband of 58 years, I convey my heartfelt gratitude for his sustained interest and generous support of my longtime involvement in the field of I&R, during which I have assumed multiple roles as a doctoral student, an I&R service provider, a university professor, and an I&R researcher and writer. Gerald's faith and confidence in me were indispensable in the completion of this book.

PART I

Introduction and Background

CHAPTER 1

I&R: Access to Human Services in an Information Era

True access demands that a citizen be offered that advice, referral or
information that comes closest to responding to his needs.
Alfred J. Kahn, 1970

BARRIERS AND IMPEDIMENTS TO ACCESS

Not knowing where to turn for information and help is a serious problem
in the United States. The average citizen often incurs great difficulty in
gaining access to needed services. Even finding information on where and
how to qualify for benefits and entitlements is often a problem. Bureaucratic
complexities, restricted admissions, extended waiting lists, and discrimi-
natory practices often pose overwhelming barriers to those in need of services. So complex and fragmented has the volume of services become that
available resources are often unknown and difficult to reach.

Even when resources are located, extended waiting lists, exclusive eligibility requirements, and other barriers may obstruct access to services.
The sheer process of application may in itself be discouraging. Extensive
and complicated application forms can be frustrating, particularly when
the language is unclear and unfamiliar to the applicant. Registering a
formal complaint or seeking legal redress for an apparent wrong or mis-
carriage of justice may prove to be overwhelming. Even the seemingly
simple act of requesting help may engender feelings of stigma and inad-
equacy and may conflict with the American ethos of self-sufficiency
and independence.

3

The literature is replete with accounts of serious consequences for the consumer that result from uncoordinated and discontinuous health and social services (Dear, 1995). Problems of access are also concerns for providers of services as reported by Cynthia C. Poindexter in her letter to the editor: "who asks: whatever happened to access? Whatever happened to being able to get a warm and trained human being on the telephone, who would offer to talk person-to-person and would be sensitive to how much courage it took to make the call in the first place?" She concludes with a recommendation that "we make our social service systems as 'user-friendly' as our computers are" (Poindexter, 1998).

To compound the problems of access, existing services may be inadequate in quality, or insufficient in quantity, or possibly too costly. For example, barriers to information on how formal systems fail to help battered women are cited as an ineffective system (Harris & Dewdney, 1994). Staff may favor selective clientele who fit their specific expertise or who have a high potential of success. Access to services may also be hampered by class and cultural disparities between service providers and consumers, often complicated by the provider's unfamiliarity with the language, customs, and cultural values of the I&R inquirer. Persons with marginal incomes, even when slightly above the prevailing poverty line, are often automatically disqualified and denied medicaid assistance with no recourse for appeal. The costs of deductibles and coinsurance payments for medicare may be prohibitive. Other less apparent costs may be entailed, such as the expense of taking time off from a job to obtain services, the costs of transportation, and possibly baby-sitting charges. But over and beyond these fiscal costs are the social costs of deprivation and helplessness.

For those who are unable to overcome these service barriers, the consequences may be disappointment, frustration, or desperation. Many inquirers tend to be shunted from one agency to another, often subjected to a "ping-pong" process of repeated referrals and ultimately documented as "closed cases." Some never succeed in reaching a helping source due to any number of impediments, including language barriers, inconvenient hours of service, and remote distances. Not knowing where to turn, whom to contact, and how to proceed, these persons remain outcasts with no opportunity to link up with available resources (Frederico, 1990).

In moving from a goods-producing economy to a service economy, the expectation is that appropriate services will be available to meet the changing social, economic, and environmental conditions that have created these needs. Despite the development of almost countless human services, however, barriers, fragmentation, and service inadequacies persist. The reality is that "our service society is overserviced but underserved." It has been noted that "the picture of social services in the United States is rather untidy; it contains numerous fragmented activities alongside overlapping provisions, all operating within jumbled networks of federal, state, and local sponsors and regulations, implemented through various methods of professional practice" (Gilbert & Specht, 1986).

As new forms of social services have emerged and have been implemented, a comprehensive picture of the complete social services network in the United States is difficult to grasp because poorly coordinated policies and disjointed administrative structures hamper efforts to carry out service programs responsibly. Many different funding sources from the public and private sectors support similar programs, and variously organized service programs often serve the same or similar client groups. Thus, a bewildering array of constantly changing regulations, guidelines, and legislative mandates has added to the planless condition and disorganization of human service systems (Reid, 1995).

INFORMATION AND REFERRAL (I&R): FACILITATING ACCESS TO SERVICES

One organizational response to help people find answers to their questions and services to meet their needs is the development of information and referral, generally referred to as I&R. Dating back to the early 1960s, I&R has evolved as a new service phenomenon that aims to facilitate access to services. The emergence of I&R during the past 40 years has closely paralleled the development of a "service society," in which services abound but access is limited. The expansion of social services since the early 1960s reflects enormous increases in the volume of services and the inclusion of expanding numbers of beneficiaries within the broad spectrum of human services (Frederico, 1990). The development of I&R is, in a sense, a response to the complexity and the unwieldedness that characterizes our planless service society. It has been noted that one of the reasons that I&R has been an almost hidden part of the human services is because I&R assumes many different names such as *First Call for Help, Help Line, and Community Information Services*. Consequently, the national Alliance of

Information and Referral Systems (AIRS) has encouraged all services that provide I&R to use the official slogan "Information and Referral: Bringing People and Services Together" (AIRS, 1995).

GOALS AND DEFINITIONS

The term "information and referral" conveys many different meanings and interpretations. There is no single, universally accepted definition of I&R, nor is there a single model that represents an ideal or a typical service. It has been observed that "though access services are becoming increasingly important in complex urban societies, they are nonetheless among the least tangible of social services" (Gilbert & Specht, 1986). This ambiguity may be due to the lack of clarity in delineating goals and defining I&R within the total spectrum of human services.

The dual goals of I&R are (a) to facilitate access to services, and (b) to overcome the many barriers that obstruct entry to needed resources. Thus, the purposes of I&R services may be defined as twofold: (a) to link the inquirer with an available, appropriate, and acceptable service, and (b) to utilize the data of an I&R reporting system for purposes of social planning, program development, outreach, advocacy, and evaluation. How these goals are carried out depends upon how I&R is defined.

Various definitions and delineations of I&R have emphasized different aspects of I&R as services, organized systems, and as networks of human services. According to the AIRS Standards (2000), "Information and Referral" is defined both as an *I&R Service* and as an *I&R System* (p. 37).

1. *Information and Referral Service:* An organization (or program within a larger organization) whose primary function is to link people in need of human services with appropriate service providers who can meet their needs. I&R services may be comprehensive covering the whole range of human services or may specialize in resources for a particular population.
2. *Information and Referral System:* A collaborative group of local comprehensive and specialized I&R services that have agreed to coordinate their resource maintenance, service delivery, publicity, and other functions to avoid duplication of effort, encourage service integration, and provide seamless access to information about community resources for people who need it.

Based on the multidimensional levels of I&R as a human service, the following comprehensive operational definition is suggested:

I&R is an organized set of systems of services, agencies, and/or networks that aims to facilitate universal access to human services. Through the use of an updated and readily retrievable resource file and/or automated databases, trained I&R staff link inquirers in need of information and/or services to appropriate resources in accordance with standards of professional practice. A reliable database also provides resources for advocacy, policy, programming, and social planning in the interest of promoting universal access to human services. (Haynes, 1995; Levinson, 1988)

In viewing the vast array of services that are provided by I&R agencies, it is essential to examine the nature and components of I&R as a professional linkage service. A glance at a list of I&R agencies indicates that I&R organizations are often identified by the specific and unique nature of the services they provide. For example, rather than using the term "information and referral services," some programs are identified as "information, referral, and follow-up services" (IRFS), thus highlighting the follow-up aspects of the service. Those agencies that are identified as information, referral, and retrieval services call attention to the technical capability of the agency to identify and retrieve information from resource files. The British term Citizens Advice Bureaus focuses on the citizen as service user and emphasizes the advice and advocacy functions of the Citizens Advice Bureaus. Community Information Centers and neighborhood information centers generally represent locality-specific information and referral services that may be associated with I&R services in local public libraries or public schools.

Because of the generalized application of the term "I&R" to many undefined service functions, it may be helpful to indicate what I&R is not. I&R is intended to be neither a clerical task nor a routine administrative intake function in a service agency. It operates as an "information-assistance" system as well as an "information-giving" service, since both the consumer and provider are involved in an interactional process. I&R requires helping skills that go well beyond the mechanics of organizing and operating a resource file. Moreover, the published inventories of resources and databases, no matter how well organized and systematically compiled, do not, in themselves, constitute an I&R service.

It should also be noted that I&R is not synonymous with information and retrieval, which is specifically designed for effective recall or extraction of information, rather than the provision of a consumer social service. Nor is I&R strictly a reference service that relies solely on published materials. Contrary to the views held by some agency personnel, I&R is not merely a screening mechanism; nor is it a routine intake procedure designed to determine whether the applicant can meet the eligibility requirements of the particular agency. Neither should I&R operate as a last resort for dead-end referrals after all prior efforts have been exhausted.

In view of the diverse population groups served by I&R, there are significant differences in the nature and delivery of I&R services. The multiple settings, varied structures, and different agency auspices under which I&R programs operate contribute to the difficulty of classifying I&R services and categorizing I&R organizations. Interestingly, the diversity in I&R programs is also reflected in the various terms that are applied to the I&R user, who is identified as the client, patient, patron, consumer, recipient, beneficiary, and inquirer; all terms that reflect differences in organizational auspices and variations in the nature of I&R services.

EXPANSION OF I&R SERVICE SYSTEMS

Since the inception of I&R in the early 1960s, I&R programs have continued to expand as freestanding agencies as well as units of existing human service organizations. Chapter 2 traces the history, growth, and development of I&R services that began as local community services but which have subsequently become operative on state, regional, and national levels, with indications of an expanding international agenda. A driving force in I&R developments during the four decades dating from the early 1960s to 2000 has been the active involvement of three national service organizations; namely, the Alliance of Information and Referral Systems, Inc., the United Way of America, and the U.S. Administration on Aging; jointly referred to as the National I&R Triad. In addition to expanding their own I&R membership programs, these three major organizations have entered into strategic alliances as they expanded their own I&R membership programs. These three organizations have also entered into strategic alliances with one another in a variety of I&R programs, thereby gaining greater impact and effectiveness in all I&R operations (see chap. 2, Table 2.1).

IMPACT OF INFORMATION TECHNOLOGY

It is apparent, however, that the most critical factor that has accelerated the expansion of I&R programs and has opened up new routes for access to human services has been the increased application of information technology within I&R service programs. The selected numbers of I&R programs that were involved in the application of information technology in the early 1980s expanded dramatically throughout the decade of the 1990s with operations ranging from local to global levels of service provision. Application of computerization within the human services succeeded in offering new opportunities to integrate social goals with technological developments that were considered unimaginable as recent as a decade ago. For example, new sources of information within the fields of human services are now available on the World Wide Web. Shared databases enable greater numbers of agencies to share information that was unavailable heretofore. Listservs permit interested persons to share, inform, and discuss subjects of mutual interest relevant to I&R operations. Telecommunications has also promoted efficient and instant communication via e-mail for both I&R providers and consumers, thus enabling the client to experience a sense of equity and empowerment. The national approval of 211 as a cost-free universal telephone number to access service is viewed as a highly significant achievement. The net result has been the creation of "new routes to human services" as illustrated in Figure 1.1.

NEW ROUTES TO HUMAN SERVICES

New routes to human service resources have been charted thanks to the capabilities of I&R to apply information technology in facilitating access to the broad fields of services that are designated to meet human needs. As noted in Figure 1.1, the selected categories of human services reflect some of the vast diversity that exists within broadly defined health and social services. There are "common human needs" that everyone experiences within a lifetime and that arise from or are created by the very structure of society (Towle, 1940). There also are "special human needs" that affect specific individuals or certain groups of individuals, which may be viewed quite differently depending on the prevailing cultural and societal norms in various eras. Whereas human needs tend to be boundless, human services are limited and often difficult to access.

Within the vast array of human services both public needs and personal

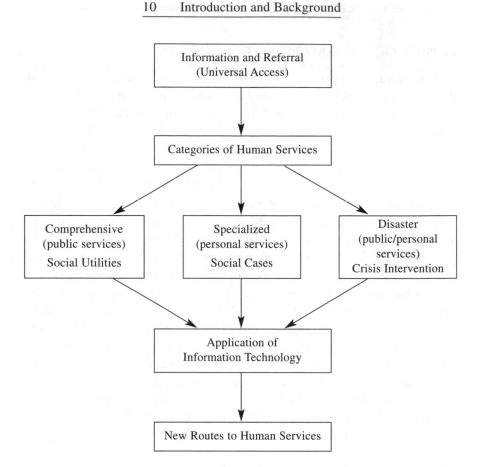

Figure 1.1 Information & Referral: New routes to human services.

needs are involved in the provision of helping services. This dual approach to the human services has been traditionally regarded as the *residual* view (personal problems) and the *institutional* view (public benefits) of social services (Wilensky & Lebeaux, 1996), depending on whether human services are needed for personal-family concerns (case services) or whether services are needed to advance the quality of life for total populations (social utilities). Whereas case services aim to provide helping services to individuals, families, and specialized groups, social utilities are directed to promote the "health and welfare" of all members of society.

In view of the unique capability of I&R services to respond to crises and disaster conditions with immediacy and with organized data on resources and helping services, a third major category of human services, which includes both individual and collective problems, has been assumed by I&R in response to emergency-crisis situations (as shown in Figure 1.1). I&R services have the capacity to be responsive to crisis and disaster situations, and have the capability to "partner" with other organizations as may be indicated. Since disasters require people to cope with chaos, shock, and at times unexpected losses, the immediacy of I&R is highly significant in responding to crisis conditions. I&R services are also involved with disaster preparedness and disaster management as are further discussed in chapters 4 and 5.

In response to these individual and collective human needs, the broad array of human services that has evolved encompasses a wide and diverse range of organized fields of services that include health and social services, income maintenance, education, housing, employment, and age-related services within the human life span that encompasses "womb-to-tomb" services. Specialized problem-related groups are involved with the concerns of disability, alcoholism, drug abuse, and criminal justice.

The enormous scope of human services can also be viewed from diverse auspices that include public, voluntary and private services, which operate within secular or sectarian agencies. Service organizations also function at a variety of different levels including local, state, regional, national, and international levels. It is important to note that service systems do not operate independently, but, in fact, tend to be interrelated, often interactive and subject to change. For example, the field of aging is dependent upon the levels of health care for older persons which, in turn, may also be dependent upon access to medical care, conditions of housing, and financial support by the existing income maintenance system. Similarly, a teenaged youth may experience such problems as addiction, a malfunctioning family, possible school problems, and perhaps even an incursion with the criminal justice system. Thus I&R manifests a multifaceted role within the diverse fields of human services.

A major turning point in "the coming of age" for I&R has been the application of information technology within operating I&R systems. The capabilities of computerization and telecommunications have brought about increased efficiencies in I&R service delivery. Computerization of resource data and service statistics has generated shared databases, new interagency alliances, and opportunities for policy formulation, research, and planning. In effect, the utilization of information technology has led to "new routes in human services" with opportunities for more effective and efficient access to human resources than has ever been possible heretofore.

Vast funds of information and access to global communication relevant to I&R services are available in the world of cyberspace. Information technology has changed many of the ways in which people interact and communicate. New opportunities to link clients to appropriate resources and new modes for case management have been greatly enhanced by applying the capabilities of technology. For I&R service providers, the World Wide Web and the Internet have facilitated access to empirical data with opportunities for data sharing and information exchange.

As noted in Figure 1.1, the modality of I&R is capable of relating to major categories of human services, which, thanks to the application of information technology, can access new routes to human services that are available via computerized operations. Through news groups, listservs, websites, online conversations, and relay chats a wealth of information can be readily obtained and shared in new and unprecedented ways (Giffords, 1998). The records of I&R agencies contain a great deal of information that can be used in a wider context for decision making and policy planning. The solution to these problems has, in the past, meant applying more scarce human resources. Over the past 40 years, however, at first slowly and subsequently, with dizzying speed, information technology is addressing problems of access as well as facilitating information exchange in the interest of problem solving and the exploration of more social choices.

Though I&R cannot provide solutions to major social problems, it can certainly assist in the identification and consideration of possible solutions, given the collective sharing of problems and informed alternatives. In the past, I&R agencies tended to be far more fragmented and more isolated, hence their databases could only be used for local purposes. The introduction of data networks in computer technology and the adoption of standardized classifications, notably the AIRS/INFO LINE taxonomy, allow for the creation of "virtual" databases that represent reported data from many I&R agencies. Appropriate analyses of shared databases can identify and track social problems and potential problems that exist beyond a local area, which may include metropolitan, state, regional, provincial, national, and international levels. By applying the capabilities of information technology, new routes to human services have been established that are capable of serving individuals, families, and communities by reaching appropriate public and private resources. I&R has increasingly developed more efficient ways for agency staff to access necessary information on behalf of their clients and in the interest of linkages with relevant resources.

DIVERSITY, ADAPTABILITY, AND NETWORKING

During the past 40 years, I&R has developed with great diversity and adaptability. I&R services operate under widely diversified varied organizational auspices in both traditional social service agencies and in many other settings such as public libraries, work sites, kiosks, and shopping malls. Comprehensive I&R programs that serve all inquirers and specialized I&R programs that are targeted to certain age groups or problem-related areas are supported by many different sources of funding from the public, voluntary, and private sectors. The vast and diverse array of providers of I&R services include (a) private, nonprofit, and profit agencies; (b) United Way voluntary action centers; (c) public libraries, schools, and hospitals; (d) city, county, and state offices; (e) military family support centers; (f) area agencies on aging; (g) child care resource and referral services; and (h) employee assistance programs (AIRS, 1997).

Service delivery is conducted by various levels of staff and may include combinations of professionals, paraprofessionals, and volunteers. The nature of I&R operations varies, depending upon whether the I&R organization is an autonomous agency or a department or unit within an established agency. I&R programs may range from an informal hot-line service to a highly sophisticated, multimillion-dollar computerized operation. I&R services may function as a telephone crisis intervention service or as a walk-in service. Organizationally, I&R may operate as a neighborhood agency, a municipal department, a regional network, a statewide system, or a federally mandated program. Because the settings and parameters of I&R systems are so varied in scope, in range of services, and in geographic service areas, an examination of the current field of I&R is vital and challenging.

The inherent diversity of I&R reflects its unique capacity to respond to current needs, opportunities, and prevailing trends with flexibility and adaptability. The impetus for the initiation of I&R services dates back to the consumerism and human rights movement of the 1960s, when the social legislation of the Older Americans Act and the antipoverty programs of the Great Society demanded new services and opportunities for access to available resources. What has contributed to the tenacity and stability of

I&R developments is an extraordinary adaptability that has sought to maximize awareness and utilization of existing resources. Rather than creating new layers of bureaucracy, I&R programs tend to rely on existing organizational structures with optimal utilization of available resources and information technology.

CONCLUSIONS

In accordance with the stated aim of AIRS in "bringing people and services together," the development of I&R has maximized linkages between persons who may need help and resources that can provide help. By applying the capabilities of information technology, I&R has demonstrated resourcefulness and pliability by creating new interagency networks and new strategies that are capable of pooling resources and sharing common tasks.

The development of widely diversified systems of I&R services, agencies, and networks, plus the dramatic developments in information technology, have opened up new routes to access services and new opportunities for innovation in service provision. To what extent can I&R service providers use this new technology in service delivery systems to provide "caring and sharing" in a society of limited resources and boundless social needs? The enormous complexity of I&R that has resulted from its extensive and uncharted growth poses new choices and challenges. Is I&R a service in itself or only a first step in the service process? If I&R is viewed as a connecting link in a caregiving chain, who links the proliferating I&R programs? Is there a need for an "I&R on I&R?" To assess the capabilities, the constraints, and the potentials of I&R, an understanding of the evolution of I&R (chap. 2) and the development of relevant information technologies (chap. 3) are a logical beginning.

REFERENCES

AIRS. (2000). *STANDARDS for professional information and referral*. Seattle, WA. AIRS.

AIRS. (1997). The many faces of information and referral. In *Information and referral: The journal of information and referral systems*. (Special Vol.). Seattle, WA: AIRS.

AIRS. (1995). *Out of the shadows—information and referral: Bringing people and services together*. Joliet, IL: AIRS.

Dear, R. B. (1995). Social welfare policy. In *Encyclopedia of social work*, (Vol. 3, pp. 2227–2234). Silver Springs, MD: National Association of Social Work.

Frederico, R. C. (1990). Why is social welfare needed? In *Social welfare in today's world* (pp. 53–73). New York: McGraw-Hill.

Giffords, E. D. (1998). Social work on the Internet: An introduction. *Social Work: Journal of the National Association of Social Workers, 43* (3), 243–253.

Gilbert, N., & Specht, H. (Eds.). (1986). *Handbook of the social services*. Englewood, NJ: Prentice Hall.

Harris, R. M., & Dewdney, P. (1994). *Barriers to information: How formal help systems fail battered women*. Westport, CT: Greenwood.

Kahn, A. J. (1970). Perspectives on access to social services. *Social Work, 15* (2), 95–101.

Haynes, K. S. (1995). Information and referral services. In *Encyclopedia of social work* (19th ed., Vol. 2, p. 1465). Washington, DC: National Association of Social Work.

Levinson, R. W. (1988). *Information and referral networks: Doorways to human services*. New York: Springer Publishing.

Levinson, R. W., & Haynes, K. S. (1984). *Accessing human services: International perspectives*. Beverly Hills, CA: Sage.

Long, N. (1973). Information and Referral services. A short history and some recommendations. *The Social Service Review, 47* (1), 49–62.

Pointdexter, C. C. (1998). Whatever happened to access? *Social Work, 43*, 383–384.

Reid, N. R. (1995). Social welfare history. In *Encyclopedia of social work*. (19th ed., Vol. 2, pp. 2206–2225). Washington, DC: National Association of Social Work.

Towle, C. (1940). *Common human needs*. New York: National Association of Social Work.

Wilensky, H., & Lebeaux, C. (1965). *Industrial society and social welfare*. (pp. 138–140). New York: The Free Press.

CHAPTER 2

Historical Perspectives on I&R

From a historical point of view, information and referral centers may be only a transitional step toward a centralized assessment and referral services for all human services.
Nicholas Long, 1973

T he genesis of access services can conceivably be traced to the origin of the human species. Had I&R services existed when Eve "referred" Adam to the Tree of Knowledge, or had there been other available information sources, the outcome for the human race might have been quite different. Though the processes of information sharing, advising, referring, and advocating are basic to all human interactional processes, formally organized I&R systems designed to facilitate access to needed resources are a relatively recent social invention of the 1960s. The following historical account of I&R developments within the four-plus decades beginning with the 1960s and continuing through to the new millennium of 2000 reflects the interests of public, private, and voluntary efforts in I&R operations under diversified auspices.

A major driving force in the continued development and expansion of I&R programs during this 40-year period has been the dynamic involvement of each of the following three national organizations: (a) the United Way of America (UWA), (b) the National Association of State Units on Aging (NASUA) under the auspices of the U.S. Administration on Aging (AoA), and (c) the Alliance of Information and Referral Systems (AIRS). However, from a historical perspective, the origins of I&R can be traced to the social service organizations that developed in the latter half of the 19th century in the United States and in Great Britain.

17

ORIGINS: EARLY I&R-TYPE PROGRAMS

A historical overview of the developments of I&R in the United States reveals an uneven and generally sporadic growth of I&R programs. The antecedents of I&R services were the Social Service Exchanges that were established by the Charity Organization Societies (COS) and the Settlement House Movement in the late 19th century (Trattner, 1994). While the COS services concentrated on helping "the poor and morally misguided persons and families," settlement houses focused on improving community life through organized services and advocacy measures. Ostensibly, the purpose of the COS exchanges was to facilitate communication among agencies to enhance service coordination; however, the real intent was to restrict access and avoid duplication of relief services (Long, 1973a). The exchanges maintained a central index of names of all recipients of cash benefits and counseling services who were known to service agencies in the community. The dual objectives of the exchanges were to prevent duplication of charitable grants to welfare recipients and to protect donors against multiple and overlapping demands. In effect, the exchanges sought to restrict rather than facilitate access to existing services.

Concurrent with the COSs were the neighborhood organizations known as settlement houses in the late 19th century, such as Hull House in Chicago in 1889 and the Henry Street Settlement House in New York in 1893. Settlement houses focused on improving local services and conducting advocacy programs aimed to improve the health and welfare of local residents in their own communities. Aware of the needs of the community and the availability of resources, settlement house workers aimed to maximize these services not only through individual referrals but primarily through community research studies, advocacy measures with local citizens, and reports to legislators. Thus, the client-focused COS and the community-based settlement houses embraced the dual commitment of I&R: to serve individuals and communities (Smith, 1995).

WORLD WAR II & I&R: CITIZEN ADVICE BUREAUS AND VETERANS INFORMATION CENTERS

Important beginnings of information and referral services occurred during and after World War II in the United Kingdom and the United States. With the onset of Germany's bombing raids on Britain in 1939, Citizens Advice

Bureaus (CABs) emerged throughout the United Kingdom under the central leadership of the National Association of Citizens Advice Bureaus (NACAB) in London. During the early 1940s, CABs were established in local communities throughout Britain and were staffed predominantly by volunteers. Throughout the war, the bureaus responded to emergency information needs related to bomb shelters, relocations, housing, and other wartime concerns. After the war, CABs remained as permanent, free-standing local service agencies available for information, advice, and advocacy (Brasnett, 1964). According to the 1993–1994 annual report of NACABs, more than 1,600 CABs are in operation throughout England, Wales, Scotland, and Northern Ireland.

In search of a model access system, Kahn and his associates studied CABs in 1966, with a view toward assessing their applicability to the U.S. scene. The CAB model was extolled for its "nonsectarian, nonpolitical, nondiscriminatory, and stigma-free" qualities. While these social policy authorities agreed that the CAB experience represents a vital and dynamic model of an organized access system, replication of the British CAB model in the United States social service system seemed neither likely nor possible. It was recommended that the United States should create its own access models through innovation and experimentation (Kahn, 1966).

America's response to the aftermath of World War II was the creation of a unique, though short-lived development of Community Advisory Centers, popularly known as Veterans Information Centers (VICs). These centers were designed to assist the returning veteran in the transition to civilian life. In 1946 more than 3,000 VICs were reported in operation under the auspices of the United States Department of Labor. The primary purpose of VICs was to provide information to the veteran on all government benefits and community services, and to make appropriate referrals for additional help. By 1948, more than 20 federal, state, and municipal agencies participated in this program. The original plan was to restrict services to a single contact, and to refer to an outside agency if an additional service was needed. The exclusionary policy of services to veterans only and the single contact policy very likely contributed to the closing of the centers by 1949. Though of brief duration, the VICs represent a significant model in the early history of U.S. I&R services and a symbol of governmental responsibility for discharged military personnel.

THE NATIONAL I&R TRIAD (THE UNITED WAY OF AMERICA, THE ADMINISTRATION ON AGING, THE ALLIANCE OF INFORMATION AND REFERRAL SYSTEMS)

The historical development of I&R services in the United States is intimately associated with the initiatives of the following three national organizations that have initiated, nurtured, and advanced I&R services and organized programs throughout the 40 years of its development: (a) UWA, (b) NASUA, under the auspices of the Administration on Aging (AoA), and (c) AIRS. In addition to the major advances that each of these organizations has made in the development and expansion of I&R, as indicated in Table 2.1 the following discussion also notes the cooperative and complementary relationships in which each of these organizations has mutually engaged with one another toward the advancement of I&R programs and services.

UNITED WAY OF AMERICA (UWA)

The number of social service exchanges that were established by the Charity Organization Societies in the late 19th century began to diminish as community welfare councils began to evolve in the early 20th century under the newly organized United Community Funds and Councils of America renamed the United Way of America (UWA) in 1970 (Brilliant, 1990). Local UWA organizations in major urban communities began developing I&R services as early as 1921. From the first community council, founded in Pittsburgh, Pennsylvania, in 1908, the number of exchanges in operation in the United States and Canada grew to 320 by 1946; however, by April 1963, the number dwindled to 97 because of a variety of reasons, including concern over confidentiality of client information and a decline in the use of the exchanges by social agencies. The Directory of Social Service Exchanges reported 40 social service exchanges in 1969, only 8 of which were also identified as information and referral centers. While the precise number of exchanges that were replaced by I&R programs is not known, there is clearly a historical link between the social service exchanges and the establishment of information and referral programs at the turn of the 20th century. Guided by UWA, community health and welfare councils began to shift from client inventories to systematized files of community resources for direct I&R services to clients. Resource files,

TABLE 2.1 A TRIAD of National I&R Service Organizations—Strategic Alliances

Organizations: Data Items	United Way of America (UWA)	Administration on Aging (AoA)	Alliance of Information & Referral Systems (AIRS)
Main offices:	Alexandria, VA	Washington, DC	Seattle, WA
Web Sites	www.unitedway.org http://national. unitedway.org	www.aoa.gov	www.airs.org
Auspices	Voluntary	Federal agency	Voluntary
Year of origin	1921	1965	1973
Units of service	Chapter affiliates	AAAs: Area agencies on aging SUAs: State units on aging	AIRS members: local, state, regional, provincial, national, and international levels
Published directory service	Where to call for help: A nationwide directory for United Way I&R services 2001	National directory for eldercare I&R 2000–2001	Directory of I&R services in the United States & Canada 1995–1996 The Electronic Directory 2001
I&R service	I&R—one of multiple services	I&R—one of multiple services	Exclusive I&R services
Technological service innovations	211, Universal access free telephone number	National telephone eldercare locator	A taxonomy-classification of human services

which served as the primary source of published community directories, were also used as grounds for decision making on budgetary allocations and community planning.

As services in the public and voluntary sectors continued to proliferate in quantity and complexity, the need for viable information and referral services became more evident to the Community Councils that emerged under the auspices of the United Way. By 1973, the first set of I&R standards and criteria for I&R was formulated by UWA. Concurrently, UWA designed one of the first service classification systems in 1973, which subsequently became a model service identification system for many I&R services throughout the United States and Canada and known as UWASIS (United Way of America Services Identification System). The basic UWA-SIS system was organized around six basic goals and included 22 service systems, 57 identified services, and 171 programs. A set of definitions for each category guided the worker in the selection of services and programs at various levels of specificity. UWASIS has subsequently been replaced by the AIRS/INFO LINE Taxonomy, as discussed in chapter 4. Through its circulating lending library, programmed manuals, training programs, and I&R roundtables, the United Way fostered educational programs for I&R directors. It is significant to note that the 1973 founding of the national AIRS organization was a spin-off of the United Way.

ADMINISTRATION ON AGING (AoA)

In accordance with the federal mandate that was stipulated under the Older Americans Act of 1965, information, referral, and assistance are required to help older people and their families in their own homes and communities. These I&R services, also identified as Information Referral and Assistance services (I&R/A) are available in the 57 State Units on Aging and in 655 local area agencies on aging. The administration of the I&R/A program is under the auspices of NASUA, which operates within the National Support Center for the Aging. AIRS and the AoA collaborated in the research study of model I&R systems in 1983. In the early 1990s, AoA supported the expense for a comprehensive ongoing bibliography on I&R under the editorship of librarians Dick Manikowski and Norman Maas.

ALLIANCE OF INFORMATION & REFERRAL SYSTEMS, INC. (AIRS)

Throughout the period of burgeoning social programs in the 1960s, there was little coordination between the diverse I&R programs that began to evolve. Roundtable sessions with directors of I&R programs were conducted under the sponsorship of the United Way at the annual National Conferences on Social Welfare. At the I&R roundtable discussions that were held at the 1970 and 1971 National Conferences on Social Welfare, I&R directors expressed an interest in developing an independent membership organization to include the broad and diversified interests that were emerging within I&R programs.

At the information and referral workshops held at the National

Conference on Social Welfare in 1972, a resolution was passed authoriz-
ing the formation of a national professional organization to be known as
the Alliance of Information and Referral Services (AIRS), that would be
available for membership to all individuals, groups, and organizations
interested in or involved in I&R. Supported initially by modest membership fees, AIRS was established in 1973 as an independent agency and
expanded rapidly under the dynamic leadership of Corazon Estava Doyle,
a social worker, who served as a volunteer executive director for 7 con-
secutive years. (Significantly, AIRS was renamed the Alliance of
Information and Referral Systems, Inc., in 1981.) After 1978, AIRS decided
to conduct its own annual conferences, independent of the National
Conferences on Social Welfare (Nance, Evans, & Smith, 1998).

AIRS currently represents a broad membership of more than 1,000 individuals, professional groups, and official I&R agencies that operate within
the public, private, and voluntary sectors. AIRS membership also includes
hot lines, self-help groups, and specialized informational services. The
1995–1996 edition of the North American AIRS Directory of I&R Services
includes the United States and Canada. An Electronic I&R Directory was
made available in 1998 with provision for continued updating. Concurrent
with its national expansion, AIRS has encouraged the development of state
and regional affiliates, which totaled 25 in the published directory of
1995–96.

AIRS has also produced and promoted a variety of publications in the
field of I&R. Annual conference proceedings, published in 1974–1977,
reflected the early organizational efforts of AIRS to establish a national
presence. AIRS currently possesses a broad membership of interested individuals, professional groups, and official I&R agencies and programs that
operate within the public, private, and voluntary sectors. Along with its
national expansion, AIRS has encouraged the development of state and
regional affiliates, which totaled 24 as of 1995. AIRS also produced and
promoted a variety of publications in the field of I&R, including the AIRs
newsletter, dating from 1975, and the AIRS journal beginning with the
first issue in 1979. Since 1992, the journal is published annually.

AIRS experienced a dramatic growth in membership with the added
affiliation of the military in all branches of the armed services. Growing
numbers of army, air force, and navy personnel are corporate members of
AIRS and seek to qualify as Certified Information and Referral Specialists
(CIRSs). Both army and navy personnel have developed military versions

of the AIRS standards and have encouraged their staff to qualify as CIRSs. Individual air force family support centers and marine corps family service centers also maintain organizational memberships in AIRS. Seventy-five military installations are listed as member agencies in the 1995–1996 AIRS directory. Chapter 5 includes a more detailed discussion on I&R in the military.

HISTORICAL HIGHLIGHTS IN I&R DEVELOPMENTS

Following is a brief overview of the development of organized I&R services over the past 40 years (1960–2000) as a relatively new and expanding social service in the vast and diversified fields of human services. Early efforts at establishing I&R services in the U.S. occurred concurrently in the public and voluntary sectors with major concern for older people as well as the economically disadvantaged and the chronically ill. Within the public sector, the federal government promoted legislation to develop locality-based I&R programs to facilitate access to community services for older people, as well as people with chronic illness or mental illness.

THE 1960S: I&R IN PUBLIC AND VOLUNTARY SECTORS

Supported by funds authorized by the Community Health Services and Facilities Act of 1961, grants were awarded to selected public and voluntary agencies to demonstrate new and improved methods of providing community health services outside the hospital, especially for people with chronic illness and older persons. The passage of the Mental Retardation Facilities and Community Mental Health Centers Act of 1963 was the landmark legislation in mental health care that advocated the relocation of mental health services from traditional state institutions to community-based facilities. Title I of the act specified information and referral, follow-up, and transportation as vital services. Title II stipulated that the comprehensive mental health center should coordinate its services with other health and social service agencies to ensure that persons receiving services within a given catchment area may have access to all health and social services.

The earliest and most extensive development of I&R services in the United States centered on older persons. Under the administration of the Older Americans Act (OAA) in 1965, and more specifically, under the Title III amendments of the OAA legislation in 1973, the AoA assumed a major leadership role in guiding the development and expansion of I&R. AoA is the only national agency in the United States with a federal mandate to establish I&R services in local, regional, and state agencies. Title III of the Older Americans Act provided matching federal grants to state-approved projects designed to deliver I&R services. Under Title IV of the act, the AoA supported a variety of large-scale research projects and special studies on I&R programs that had significant impact on I&R developments for older persons as well as for all population groups. The 1973 amendments to the OAA strongly recommended networking of I&R with other community agencies to promote effective, coordinated services to older persons (See chap. 6 on aging).

I&R services were also suggested for the economically disadvantaged groups in the diverse social programs of the 1960s. To meet the needs of the economically deprived, Title II-A of the Economic Opportunity Act of 1964 created quasi-public community action programs (CAPs) for service delivery to the local persons with low income. This legislation specified the provision of information and referral services, along with transportation, outreach, follow-up, legal services, and escort services. However, since the antipoverty programs were directed to the most economically deprived groups in the community, I&R tended to be restricted to the local community action programs for persons with low income. Nevertheless, the leaders in the antipoverty programs, who were strong advocates for consumer rights, also called attention to the need for universal access to community services, beyond the needs of the economically disadvantaged.

The establishment of I&R-type programs in national voluntary health organizations occurred concurrently with I&R developments in the social programs of the 1960s. As early as 1913, the American Red Cross (ARC) incorporated aspects of I&R services into its home care program for the sick and infirm. By 1918, Red Cross workers began to receive I&R training in information giving, referral, and follow-up techniques in disaster-aid programs. Operationally, the ARC has endorsed the principle of collaboration with other I&R programs that operate in health and social agencies for the purpose of facilitating access to services for the civilian population as well as for military personnel. Traditionally, the ARC has responded with crisis intervention programs, including I&R-type services to provide emergency aid under catastrophic conditions (Tannenbaum, 1981).

In 1962 the National Easter Seal Society for Crippled Children and Adults began a self-study that concluded that I&R services should be conducted by all affiliates of the national organization to help people with disabilities live purposeful lives through the effective use of available resources. For those communities in which I&R centers were not already in operation, local Easter Seal chapters took the initiative to provide I&R services concurrently with specialized services for people with disabilities.

In a joint effort to establish guidelines and basic criteria for the rapidly emerging I&R programs that began in the 1960s, Bloksberg and Caso (1967) conducted the first comprehensive national survey of I&R services under the cosponsorship of the United States Public Health Service and the Florence Heller Graduate School for Advanced Studies in Social Welfare at Brandeis University. Of 269 information and referral centers that were included in this study, more than half (151) reported specialized I&R programs for older persons and I&R services related to health and mental health problems, particularly alcoholism. The remaining I&R programs (118) identified their programs as generic. The survey findings highlighted the need for continued research and evaluation and anticipated the rapid expansion of I&R that occurred in the 1970s.

THE 1970S: RESEARCH, NEW CLIENTELE, AND SETTINGS

The 1970s marked a period of rapid growth of I&R service organizations. New free-standing I&R agencies emerged concurrently with I&R units and departments that developed within existing health and social service agencies. A mounting interest in universal service provision suggested the need for more generic I&R services. Consequently, broader population groups became the beneficiaries of I&R services, and I&R programs emerged in new and nontraditional settings.

Research

During the 5-year period from 1969 to 1974, the AoA also sponsored a series of working papers and research studies conducted by Nicholas Long of Interstudy Associates, a research organization located in Minneapolis. Long developed an extensive series of working papers published by Interstudy (1974) on specific skills and techniques involved in I&R program development and aspects of service delivery, including information giving and referral, interviewing, follow-up, and outreach. Long's functional analysis of the 1967 survey by Bloksberg and Caso provided a valuable interpretation of the impact of I&R and highlighted the capability of

I&R to serve as a valuable social planning resource. An evaluative study of the Wisconsin I&R system conducted by Long and his associates during the early 1970s set a precedent for evaluative research in I&R networking (Long, 1973b). Under Long's leadership an extensive annotated bibliography on I&R was published in 1972 that reflected an early state-of-the-art report on I&R.

New Clientele

The human-rights movement that was initiated in the 1960s continued to generate new demands for services in the 1970s and identified new groups of users, including people with disabilities, the unemployed, women, and children. Although special programs for people with disabilities were included in the Social Security Act of 1935, minimal provision for access to services was available until the decade of the 1970s, which Bruck (1978) called "the decade of disability." The implementation of the Education for All Handicapped Children Act of 1975 required the "mainstreaming" of children with disabilities in public school programs and optimal utilization of resources in the integration of the handicapped into existing community service programs. The Bill of Rights Act of 1975 for the Developmentally Disabled (PL 94–103) clearly specified "maximum development under the least restrictive conditions." Formally organized advocacy programs, as well as informal self-help programs organized by and for people with disabilities, indicated the need for access to generic as well as specialized services. To promote the Independent Living Programs for people with disabilities, The Information Center of Hampton Roads, Virginia, developed a specialized program of I&R services for the disabled within their generic program of services. On a national level, the United States Clearinghouse on the Handicapped was concurrently engaged in the compilation and dissemination of information and the promotion of advocacy for people with disabilities.

The proliferation of hot lines and self-help groups represented a diversified range of special interest groups in need of information, referral, and advocacy to serve the special interests of single parents, abused women, persons with disabilities, ethnic minorities, and other interest groups. Self-help groups have also emerged on college campuses to staff hot lines and drop-in services and provide information and peer counseling on a person-to-person basis.

To meet child care needs for working parents, growing numbers of corporations have developed a variety of I&R programs. Some of these child care programs operate on company sites; others function as resource referring organizations for child care. A growing trend has been to help parents locate satisfactory child care within their own communities through referral and collaboration with available and appropriate child care programs. The major motivation for the support of I&R day care services by corporations has been to reduce employee absenteeism and promote productivity. I&R developments in child care reflected the increased involvement of the private sector in social welfare services since public day care services are limited and the volume of working mothers has increased. For growing numbers of profit-making organizations, I&R is a significant employee benefit that operates in the interest of "good business."

New Settings

A shift toward universal I&R programs at all levels of operation was reflected in the implementation of Title XX of the Social Security Act in 1974. The public provision of I&R for all citizens and "not for the poor alone" created a trend toward increased centralization of I&R systems at state and regional levels. The availability of Title XX funds for I&R program development and I&R training contributed to the rapid expansion of I&R services that far surpassed I&R developments prior to the 1970s. By 1981, almost all states reported a level of I&R services, although the actual amounts allocated by each state for I&R varied enormously. In view of the options offered under Title XX, some states chose not to operate their own I&R systems but to contract with I&R services that operated outside of the public sector. Thus, an important precedent for public-voluntary partnerships in I&R service delivery was established.

The expansion of I&R in the 1970s occurred not only within traditional social agencies but also extended to nontraditional settings, such as public libraries. The informational role of the library was extended whereby the public library could serve both as a local information center and a direct service center. The earliest experiment in library-based I&R programs was conducted in 1969, when the Enoch Pratt Free Library Service in Baltimore collaborated with the Library School at the University of Maryland to operate the Public Information Center. Despite its limitations, due to inadequate staff and insufficient top-level administrative support, the Public Information Center set a notable precedent of a library-based I&R service until its close in 1973 (Donohue, 1976). Unlike Maryland's limited I&R program, the Detroit Public Library established an I&R service in 1971 known as The Information Place (TIP) that involved the total library staff in the training and delivery of I&R services. Regarded as a priority service by the library administration, The Information Place became a model I&R service for public libraries and has continued to be an innovative library program in the field of I&R (see chapter 5 on public libraries).

In 1972 the first professional conference on information and referral services in public libraries was held at the University of Illinois. The issue that called forth a heated debate was whether I&R is a professional library service or a casework service for professional social workers. A major federally funded project designed to study the effectiveness of library-based I&R services was the Urban Neighborhood Information Centers Project that was conducted during a 3-year period, from 1972 to 1975, in five major cities (Atlanta, Cleveland, Detroit, Houston, and Queens Borough, New York). While I&R programs developed differently in each of these urban sites, the project made a significant impact by demonstrating that the public library can effectively serve as a community information center and thereby expand its services far beyond the reference file (Puryear, 1982). Since 1971, the American Library Association has recognized I&R as an important user-oriented service and has designated I&R as a vital goal for all public library services.

Another new setting that has assumed a growing importance for I&R programs since the early 1970s is the workplace. Labor unions traditionally sought to meet members' needs through the development of social services programs that were concerned with personal services. Wary of the formally organized social welfare agencies and suspicious of involvement with the formal social welfare community, organized labor's go-it-alone philosophy led to the development of informal networks of I&R-type services that were operated by individual union leaders who functioned as advocates, using a family support approach to assist union members with their problems both at and outside the work site.

Formal union programs have subsequently developed in which social workers are hired to deliver I&R services or to train rank-and-file worker-volunteers to serve as information and referral agents at the work site. Various other union programs operate in combination with established social welfare agencies that provide I&R services. To provide I&R training to company personnel, the UWA initiated a referral agent program in

1974 in which selected company employees were trained to serve as I&R agents within their own organizations. In the corporate sector, a growing number of Employment Assistance Programs have assumed the responsibility of providing I&R services in the workplace.

THE 1980S: NEW PARTNERSHIPS AND ALLIANCES

The need for improved coordination became increasingly evident by the 1980s when growing number of agencies continued to expand I&R programs without guidelines and planned coordination. In the face of service cutbacks and major reductions in budgetary allocations, I&R agencies attempted to minimize the negative effects of diminishing social services by maximizing access to services and creating new partnerships with other service agencies, thereby promoting interorganizational collaborations.

The 1980s also initiated a growing involvement of the private corporate sector such as the American Telephone and Telegraph Company (AT&T). Directories of toll-free telephone numbers published by AT&T, as well as new nationwide pricing plans for instate long-distance calling, have expanded telephone communications, which, in turn, have had implications for I&R operations. In addition to designing new products to meet the special communications needs of people with disabilities, AT&T has also collaborated with other agencies to set up consumer telephone hot-lines to answer questions and facilitate access to information and needed resources.

THE 1990S: IMPACT OF TECHNOLOGY

A major factor in the expansion of I&R networks in the 1980s and 1990s has been the rapid advances in automation that have produced unprecedented capabilities in communications and intersystems linkages. As computers became far more affordable during the early 1990s, increasing numbers of agencies replaced manual files with computers and sought suitable classification systems to organize their data files. Centralization of shared databases for systematic access, storage, and retrieval has enhanced the selection and management of voluminous funds of data within interactive information systems.

Taxonomy: A New Service Classification

Among the most dramatic developments in I&R that occurred throughout the decade of the 1990s was the expanding development of a new classification system known as the INFO LINE, LA Taxonomy, and the gains in professionalism relevant to I&R services. INFO LINE was developed by the Federation of Social Agencies of Los Angeles under the leadership of Georgia Sales and rapidly gained recognition as an effective thesaurus for the field of I&R. By 1997, the AIRS organization endorsed the INFO LINE Taxonomy as the standard classification system. UWA followed with its endorsement in 1998. AIRS/INFO LINE has gained broad acceptance as an effective data-reporting system, and is, in fact, regarded as a first step in the development of a common language for the identification of social service categories. Concurrent with the development of AIRS/INFO LINE, there has been a parallel development in the design of software systems.

211 Universal Telephone Access

A highly important innovation that began in the late 1990s has been the establishment of the universal toll-free telephone number, 211, as a nationally approved community service by the Federal Communications Center. In 1997 the United Way of Atlanta created the nation's first three-digit telephone number which connects callers to the full array of community resources within local communities and beyond. United Way 211 in Atlanta is a free, 24-hour telephone I&R service. Using a database of over 2,000 agencies, it matches callers to social services and to volunteer opportunities and donation sources. In 1999 Connecticut began using 211 as the statewide access point for residents to link with local public and private health and social services. According to an executive summary regarding the national 211 Initiative to Link People with Community Resources submitted on April 27, 2000 by Peter Aberg, executive director of AIRS, the Atlanta and Connecticut 211 services each receive approximately 200,000 calls per year. Groups in 41 other states were concurrently involved in efforts to implement 211 for community service purposes. It should be noted that every area customizes the 211 service to address local needs with other N11 numbers such as 911. Chapter 3 includes a more extended discussion on 211.

ADVANCES IN I&R PROFESSIONALISM

Comparable to the process of professionalization in other human service organizations, AIRS was initiated primarily as a volunteer-operated social service. With growing local, state, and regional I&R operations, formal recognition of I&R service providers and acceptance of accredited organizations became important for public recognition and for funding qualifications. As AIRS continued to expand and gain recognition the need for professionalization became more urgent. As a process that generally occurs within the maturation of a social service, volunteerism tends to be supplanted by professionalism, a process which entails approved standards, a code of ethics, organizational accreditation and certified personnel. AIRS took the initiative to formalize the requirements for professionalism and gained recognition and approval from UWA and subsequently from AoA, as members of the I&R TRIAD.

The most dramatic gains that I&R made in professionalism were realized during the decade of the 1990s. The fourth edition of the AIRS standards was published in the year 2000 as the official body of "standards for professional I&R." These standards present an updated report on essential functions of I&R service delivery, data collection systems, multilevel networking, and organizational requirements (See Appendix E–Summary of I&R Standards).

Professional advances in I&R occurred when AIRS arrived at a formal procedure for certification, which enabled I&R providers to gain recognition as *professionals* in the field of I&R. A formal application and subsequent exam have enabled I&R providers to qualify as professional certified staff. AIRS also instituted a formal process for I&R organizations to acquire accreditation based on meeting specific criteria to gain professional recognition. A formal procedure of certification under the auspices of AIRS enabled I&R providers to gain recognition as CIRS. Further description of each of these professional attainments is discussed in chapter 8.

INTERNATIONAL REPORT ON I&R

The increasingly wider application of automation by growing numbers of I&R agencies has promoted broader networks and interactive communication among I&R systems. Information technology has permitted the sharing of data and interactive communication on an international basis. As previously noted, Kahn and his associates singled out the CAB model as worthy of consideration as a universal access system. However, acknowledging that no composite or ideal model of an access system exists, Kahn advised that the United States must try to "experiment" with local social service centers and find its own appropriate model. In the United States, there is no parallel to the hierarchical levels of organization that operate within the CAB system in the United Kingdom. Local CABs are governed by their own management committees and are responsible to regional area committees, which, in turn, are accountable to the central office of NACABs in London.

Both the British CABs and U.S. I&R models have influenced the organization of access systems in other developed and developing countries. In those countries that have had an association with the British Commonwealth (e.g., Australia, India, Israel, and South Africa), access systems have tended to follow the CAB pattern of operation. In a 1984 study, Levinson & Haynes reported that the unique and innovative features of access systems in Cyprus, Japan, and Poland reflected the idiosyncratic nature of their respective social welfare systems. In all the reported access systems under study, the role of the volunteer was prominent. In addition to a focus on consumer-centered services, these cross-national reports emphasized the capabilities of access systems which contribute to social planning, policy formulation, and social reform.

Considering Canada's physical proximity to the United States, and given the funding supplied by UWA to Canadian agencies, Canadian I&R systems tend to resemble the U.S. I&R model. The Information Canada Federation, which was incorporated as a national not-for-profit organization in June 2000 represents a regional member of AIRS (Evans, 2000). The Canada-wide information and referral organization is known as InformCanada. According to Gil Evans, two major projects that have been undertaken are the Toronto Human Service Information System and the Calgary Health And Social Services Information System. The Toronto Human Service Information System is a single comprehensive information utility that will consolidate all human services information in Toronto— and potentially other jurisdictions. The InformCanada web site (www.info. london.on.ca/informcanada/) includes a list of all operating I&R services in Canada (Evans, April 2000). On August 9, 2001, *the Canadian Radio-Television and Telecommunications Commission* (CRTC) reserved 211 for the exclusive use of community information and referral (Jones).

An international invitation was extended to AIRS by Community Information Victoria and the Australian Community Networking Alliance to attend Australia's Premier Networking Conference held on September 29, 1999. Speakers were described as "networking leaders" from Australia, New Zealand, the United Kingdom, and the United States. It was also noted that Civic, Victoria's community information agency, produced its own

Community Information Thesaurus to provide "a common indexing language for information needs."

Another vital aspect of international I&R is the involvement of the military in I&R programs that operate throughout the world. Increased numbers of military attend the annual AIRS training conferences, and growing numbers of I&R military personnel are qualifying as CIRS. (See chapter 5 on military I&R).

CONCLUSIONS

To understand I&R, one must take into account the recency and rapidity of the development and expansion of this social service. While origins of I&R-type programs have been traced to the social services exchanges of a century ago, I&R services are essentially a product of the 1960s that became institutionalized in I&R organizations during the 1970s and generated expanding I&R networks in the 1980s. The 1990s provided a new decade of explosive growth of I&R programs and new strategic alliances. The expansion of I&R services in the 1990s has been the result of the enormous impact of information technology and the development of shared databases. Professionalization of I&R was strongly promoted with the publication of new standards in 2000, the certification of I&R specialists, the accreditation of I&R agencies, a universal taxonomy, and the initiation of the universal 211 telephone number. Chapter 3, which follows, provides a historical background on the development and expansion of information technology as it relates to the field of I&R.

REFERENCES

Bloksberg, L. M., & Caso, E. K. (1967). *Survey of information and referral services existing within the U.S.: Final report*. Waltham, MA: Brandeis University, Florence Heller Graduate School of Advanced Studies in Social Welfare.

Brasnett, M. E. (1964). *The story of the Citizen's Advice Bureau*. London: The National Council of Social Service.

Brilliant, E. L. (1990). *The United Way: Dilemma of organized charity* (p. 40). NY: Columbia University Press.

Bruck, L. (1978). *Access—The guide to a better life for disabled Americans*. New York: Random House-David Obst Books.

Donohue, J. C. (1976). The public information center project. In M. Kochen, & J. D. Donohue (Eds.), *Information for the community* (pp. 79–93). Chicago: American Library Association.

Evans, G. (2000, April). Report from the Great White North. *AIRS Newsletter: Alliance of Information and Referral Systems, 24* (2), 18.

Evans, G. (2000, August). Report from the Great White North. *AIRS Newsletter: Alliance of Information and Referral Systems, 24* (4), 17.

Interstudy. (1974). *Information and referral services: Interviewing and information giving.* Minneapolis: Institute for Interdisciplinary Studies of the American Rehabilitation Foundation. (ERIC Document Reproduction Service No. ED 055 635).

Jones, C. (2001, October). Approved in Canada. *AIRS Newsletter–Alliance of Information and Referral Systems.* pp. 4–5.

Kahn, A. J., Grossman, L., Bandler J., Clark, F. R., Galkin, F., & Greenwalt, K. (1966). *Neighborhood information centers: A study and some proposals.* New York: Columbia University School of Social Work.

Long, N. (1973a). Information and referral services. A short history and some recommendations. *The Social Service Review, 47* (1), 49–62.

Long, N. (1973b). *Wisconsin information service, an I&R Network.* Wisconsin Division on Aging, Department of Health and Social Services. (September 1973).

Nance, W., Evans, G., & Smith, H. (1998). *AIRS: The first 25 years (1973–1998).* Seattle, WA: AIRS.

Puryear, D. (1982). Early I&R programs in libraries. *Information and Referral: The Journal of the Alliance of Information and Referral Systems, 4* (2), 16–20.

Smith, R. F. (1995). Settlements and neighborhood centers. In *Encyclopedia of Social Work* (19th ed., Vol. 3, p. 2129). Washington, DC: NASW.

Tannenbaum, M. A. (1981). I&R in the American Red Cross: A collaborative program. *Information and Referral: The Journal of the Alliance of Information and Referral Systems, 3* (1), 37–47.

Trattner, W. I. (1994). *From poor law to welfare state: A history of social welfare in America.* (5th ed.). New York: The Free Press.

CHAPTER 3

I&R: Coming of Age in an Information Revolution

Cyberspace is not a cold universe of bits and bytes—
but a rich warm world full of people who connect and
share and care for each other.
Tom Ferguson, 1996

INTRODUCTION: THE DIGITAL SOCIETY

There is a profound change underway in the ability of ordinary citizens to communicate with one another and to access information that helps in the solution of problems in everyday living. It is the new information technologies, particularly the Internet and the World Wide Web that are providing the infrastructure and tools that drive this revolution. The development of information and referral services during the past 40 years has occurred concurrently with the enormous advances in information technology that have impacted all dimensions of living, including the human services. New developments in communications have brought about worldwide networks of computers through which ordinary citizens bank and make travel reservations for hotels, airlines, and rental cars, all from the comfort of their homes. Computer networks link information systems that have the ability to share information with unprecedented speed and effectiveness.

Distance education, distance medicine, and distance shopping over real-time computer networks are becoming boom industries. More and more people are "banking" and implementing investment decisions from home. Dispersed families and friends are staying in touch with one another through electronic mail and interactive chat sessions—sessions that are beginning

37

to use two-way video as well as audio. Students are "attending" college courses without leaving their homes and physicians are making diagnoses of diseases in patients they have never seen. All manner of people are able to use digital information technologies for access to information that can help to solve everyday problems. Information service agencies such as libraries and I&R agencies are finding that access to digital resources advances their ability to provide helpful information to clients. A major benefit of networked computer databases is that they can offer around-the-clock accessibility for people who need information at times convenient for them.

Electronic mail (e-mail) and electronic discussion groups have dramatically expanded professional communication. Professionals of all kinds are "talking" with one another through these technologies in order to share common problems and to assist one another in their solution. Geographic distance has become much less of a barrier to professional communication. Along with professionals in other fields, I&R service professionals nationwide are adopting these new technologies. For example, the *i-r listserv* (an electronic discussion group for I&R workers) is extremely active and is an invaluable channel for information and problem sharing. I&R service providers are adopting information technologies for essentially the same reasons as other professionals—to manage their internal systems more efficiently, to provide a higher level of services to clients, and to facilitate communications and resource sharing among individuals in different institutions.

As computers have become more affordable and more manageable for the uninitiated, and as information systems have become increasingly user-friendly, the utilization of computers in industry, government, and social services, as well as in the home, has created an unprecedented information revolution that has also impacted I&R developments:

Data, information, and knowledge are often used interchangeably, but they are not the same. Data are the raw material produced by observation or measurement; information results from processing of data into its relevant, useful, and meaningful components. Data are facts and information that are necessary for some purpose and that have meaning and significance. Knowledge results from the processing of information into a coherent body of facts. Knowledge can be viewed as a collection of information which can be used to generate new data and information. (Geiss & Viswanathan, 1986)

THE EARLY YEARS: THE 1950s

How did we arrive at this information revolution? At the heart of today's information technologies is the digital computer. Digital computers were developed during the 1940s as part of the national defense effort. These computers were cumbersome, extremely expensive, and had no application beyond mathematical computation. In the early 1950s digital computers were found only in defense establishments and a few research laboratories. The invention of the transistor in the early 1950s led to the development of the first transistorized computer in 1956. The transistor was an essential element in advancing the technical development of computers so that the late 1950s saw the introduction of far more reliable and cheaper digital computers for use in government and in the corporate sector. Smaller organizations that could not afford the cost of a mainframe computer rented time in computer bureaus. In essence, these early commercial computers were used for tabulation tasks that had previously been done by clerks with adding machines or with other mechanical tabulation devices. Use of computers as tools for manipulating and accessing textual information, such as resource databases, was in its infancy.

MOVING INTO THE MAINSTREAM: THE 1960s

The 1960s saw the beginnings of computer use for storing and manipulating textual data for publication in print format and later for direct access. Information agencies such as large academic and public libraries used computers to publish printed catalogs of their collections. The abstracting and indexing services of scholarly societies such as the American Psychological Association pioneered the use of computers to publish their indexes to journal literature. Once such data were in digital format (usually on magnetic tapes) it was a logical step for these organizations to go beyond print on paper by providing direct terminal access to their databases. By the late 1960s with the creation of services such as Dialog, dozens of digital databases became available, the U.S. National Library of Medicine's Medline online database, one of the major sources for biomedical literature dates from this period. Computers of the 1960s were large mainframe computers that required special environments in which to operate. The rooms that housed these machines had to be air-conditioned and required special electrical wiring. Computer applications were not run by end users but required the intervention of highly trained data processing personnel. The cost of a mainframe computer ranged from several hundred thousand to several million dollars and the ongoing operating costs were also high.

THE GOLDEN YEARS: THE 1970s

The 1970s were, in many respects, the golden years for the adoption and use of computer technologies. The falling price of hardware together with the introduction of minicomputers made it possible for smaller organizations to consider introducing computer applications. Uses expanded to automation of many labor-intensive activities within organizations. In the information field, direct, real-time access to digital databases became routine in the academic and research world. Among the larger I&R agencies that had access to the still-expensive computer technologies, some interesting projects were undertaken. For example, the I&R system operated by the United Way of Texas Gulf Coast is an example of an effective data-retrieval system that used I&R data for planning purposes. In 1976 this agency established an automated data system using a machine-readable client case log form. The I&R system maintained a sophisticated online retrieval program on an IBM mainframe that was accessed via in-house terminals. Workers completed one form for each I&R call, indicating the following information for each direct service transaction: name, address, telephone number, race, age, and sex of the client; problems encountered; referrals processed; time spent on referrals; and follow-up action. These computer-ready forms were completed by filling out various blanks on the inquiry form, after which the forms were read by an optical scanner. A variety of monthly reports were produced that included the number of calls by problem areas, number of cases referred to specific agencies, demographic data, and follow-up on referrals that included agencies referred to, actions taken, and documentation of unmet needs. Recognizing that computerized I&R databases could potentially have applications that go beyond service provision, some in the field began to call for the use of these systems for identification of needs and for social planning (Haynes & Sallee, 1979).

However, even I&R agencies that realized the potential for introducing computer technologies at this time faced major obstacles. Sullivan (1979) pointed out that both software developers and training centers shared a business-oriented attitude and largely ignored the special needs of I&R agencies. Data processing professionals were comfortable creating software for typical business applications but were reluctant to learn what was for them a new environment, namely, I&R. Purchase of computers was considered by organizations with an annual operating budget of at least $500,000 (in 1979 dollars). The high cost of these systems prohibited even large I&R agencies from owning their own computers, and access to computers for them meant time-sharing on the computers owned by others.

MINIATURIZATION OF INFORMATION TECHNOLOGIES: THE 1980s

The many seminal developments of the earlier decades reached fruition in the 1980s with the introduction and rapid adoption of the personal computer (PC) and the development of the Internet, as we know it today. Much of the computing that takes place in organizations today, including I&R agencies, is done on networked microcomputers, a trend that was established during the 1980s. It is not surprising that this decade saw the appearance of literature on computer applications in I&R agencies. The AIRS Newsletter (March–June 1983) reported the following: "'Home Computer: Boon or bane?' a seminar for human service professionals and others by the American Home Economics Association, San Francisco, July 29–31." The newsletter also reported an announcement of a list of free public domain software and also included tips on implementing a computerized management information system as well as a review of the Computer Resource Guide for Nonprofits.

During the 1960s and 1970s a number of I&R agencies adopted microfilm/fiche technologies for data storage and retrieval. By the 1980s the shortcomings of this technology were beginning to be recognized and an alternative was seen in computer technology. I&R agencies with microform records began to migrate to computers. For example, with the help of outside funding, First Call Minnesota transferred the agency's resource file, volunteer opportunities file, and client data from a microfiche system to an online system.

The introduction of computer technology in social agencies encouraged the development of specialized software. For example, the development and implementation at the University of Texas Medical Branch of a computer-assisted case management program reported that the Medicare's Prospective Payment System forced "sicker" patients with limited resources to more quickly return to their home communities (Wimberley, Blazyk,

Crawford, & Hokanson, 1987). Because of the growing availability of the IBM PC and its clones, some I&R software vendors whose products were designed for larger mainframes and minicomputers began to develop new versions of their software for the PC market. For example, while Active Software of Minneapolis was still developing new versions of its I&R Assistant, software for larger systems such as the IBM 38 and 36, were also rewriting the system for use on IBM PCs that would support several users over a local area network.

SPECIALIZED SOFTWARE

Specialized I&R database software allowed users access to information for a variety of needs and from different viewpoints. The data could generally be searched according to any of the following: by name of the agency, by type of service category, by geographic locations, or by keyword. Each agency, program, or service facility could also be accessed under an established service identification system, with code numbers assigned to identify the service program as well as the specific agency that offered the particular service. The purpose of geographical access was to allow the inquirer to identify resources that were available at a convenient location for the inquirer. Varying geographical and jurisdictional units are used to specify service locations, depending upon the boundaries of defined service areas. Census tract data were especially useful to correlate client data with recorded socioeconomic and demographic data extracted from federal census reports. For purposes of standardized reporting, I&R service areas could also be organized according to postal zip codes, school districts, health-planning areas, geographical boundaries, or jurisdictional divisions.

Not all I&R agencies were new to computerization. A growing number had gained considerable experience with computer systems and, by the 1980s, were ready to replace their existing systems with newer and better systems. Sherman (1986) discussed the need for agencies with outdated computer systems to upgrade to more powerful systems that would allow these agencies to offer better and more efficient services than was possible before. Sherman challenged agencies to use their computing resources for more than printing Rolodex cards. He advocated computers with capabilities to maintain bulletin boards and to handle statistical data.

Awareness of and interest in the use of digital information technologies among I&R agencies was evident at the 1984 California AIRS Conference which held, as part of its program, a workshop entitled "The Electronic

Connection" and included exhibits of computer hardware and software. In the same year, the U.S. Bureau of National Affairs announced that it would be offering many of its publications in digital form as electronic databases. However, during the 1980s, computers were really not "user-friendly," and it required considerable training to use one effectively and efficiently. I&R professionals seemed to be acutely aware of this and the need for highly user-friendly systems that required little training. Vanderheiden (1989) described an "ultra" user-friendly database for information and referral along with the principles for its development. Interestingly, the design was based on a metaphor, the printed book. The system was developed for use on Macintosh computers, whose operating system was recognized at the time as being highly user-friendly.

PROBLEMS IN EARLY I&R DIGITAL SYSTEMS

The introduction of computer technology did not go smoothly for all I&R agencies. Indeed, there were some notable failures and valuable lessons learned. The reported experiences of various I&R programs reflect some of the difficulties encountered by I&R agencies in implementing and operating automated systems. The Community Service Planning Council in Philadelphia became involved with computerization in the early 1970s and initially attempted to make an online computer system available for the I&R services of Philadelphia. Although more than $1 million was spent on this effort, the system never became operational. A major problem was that the computer program that needed to be tested and debugged by the computer consultant was not completed before the funding resources were exhausted. The shared administrative structure also posed a potential hazard, since this project was jointly administered by the Community Service Planning Council and the United Way of southern Pennsylvania. The dual organizational structure under which this project was administered did not facilitate timely decision making, thereby further impeding the implementation of this overambitious undertaking (Garrett, 1984).

Various I&R systems have encountered problems of computerization because of the lack of well-trained staff and managers for their automated systems. Insufficient political support is another major reason why computerized I&R systems became defunct, as was the experience of the Wisconsin Network, following the termination of federal funds. The ambitious planning study of the Citizens' Urban Information Centers, which was designed for 187 library-based I&R programs in New York City branch libraries, was never implemented owing to political strife and dissension that prevailed during the early 1970s (Puryear, 1982).

LESSONS LEARNED

By the mid-1980s some valuable lessons had been learned with regard to computer applications in I&R agencies. The early implementation of automated systems in the human services demonstrated that computer technology could promote greater administrative efficiency through use of management information systems (MISs). In I&R operations, data on services provided client characteristics, client eligibility, case dispositions, and budgetary allocations could be systematically entered into MIS programs and retrieved for a variety of managerial purposes. MIS data proved useful for planning programs and evaluating services. An added capability was the possibility of cross-tabulating service statistics with available sociodemographic data on client characteristics, such as specific age groups, income levels, ethnic groups, and housing conditions within designated geographical areas.

Perhaps the most widely acknowledged capability of I&R programs was the production of service inventories, which, through automation, could produce specialized directories from specific sections of the master working file or database. For example, the I&R system in the San Mateo, California, county library published a directory that contained about half of all entries in the master file; in Colorado Springs, the public library offered a complete printout of all entries in any requested portion of the total resource file. In Ontario, Canada, community information databases and networks were developed using an interactive videotext system that allowed the user to select "pages" of electronically transmitted text for viewing on a standard television set. This videotext system, known as Telidon, permitted its users to interact with a master resource database and allowed the transmission of text and the display of graphics using a telephone network with viewing capabilities added to the home color television set. Telidon was used by the Toronto Federation of Community Information Centers to create its own databases related to local user needs (Bellamy & Forgie, 1984).

An exceedingly helpful capability of I&R systems was the monitoring and inventorying of available resources through automated vacancy programs. In 1974–1975, Philadelphia developed an online computerized service registry designed to provide up-to-date, accurate information on vacancies in day care programs, nursing homes, and low-income housing. A client could inquire about any one of these services, indicate preferred locations, and receive information on the level of fees and the mode of payment that was acceptable (e.g., Medicaid or Medicare). Based on the client's specifications, a list of agencies with available openings could then be generated. The Service Opening Registry, established in Philadelphia in 1974, was updated at least weekly, but was abandoned because the maintenance and updating costs proved to be extremely high and exceeded the fiscal limits of the agency's funds (Levinson, 1988).

Unlike the Philadelphia vacancy program, which assumed total responsibility for maintaining updated inventories, the Crisis Clinic in Seattle relied upon the initiatives of interested service agencies for reports on their current inventories. The basic resource file could be modified to serve as a tracking system for vacancies in day care and shelter facilities. Staff at area day care centers and shelters bore the responsibility of informing the clinic when openings occur. Data on space openings were entered into the system and automatically removed after 1 week, thereby providing continued tracking and updating with minimal monitoring costs on the part of the I&R agency. The data retrieval system for this vacancy inventory was programmed to yield information on clientele, hours, fees, and geographic locations.

An area that attracted increased attention in I&R operations was the application of decision support systems (DSSs) as an aid for professional assessments and case planning. A DSS is an interactive, flexible, and adaptive information system developed to support a nonstructured management problem for improved decision making. This system utilizes data, provides an easy user interface, and allows for the decision maker's own insights. The goals of a DSS are to facilitate high decision quality, the creation of new insights and learning, and improved management decisions. Diagnosing clients and designing treatment plans based on computerized data became a new but growing element in I&R operations. Computers had proved their importance in medical and clinical practices as helpful aids in arriving at medical diagnoses and treatment alternatives.

By the close of the 1980s there was recognition, at least among the I&R leadership, that changes in how agencies conduct their business due to increased use of computers was inevitable. It was believed that electronic applications of services would finally force the various I&R players in our respective communities to work for greater coordination. Automation would force referral providers in close proximity to one another to answer a very basic question: Why aren't you supporting a commonly shared database?

DEMOCRATIZATION OF INFORMATION: THE 1990S

A striking trend in computer technology for the decade of the 1990s was the move from centralized computing systems to distributed client server computer systems connected by networks. An important effect of this change is the reduced level of expertise required to interact with computer systems. Development and maintenance of information systems based on centralized mainframe or mini computers was an esoteric task that required highly trained technical staff. The distributed computer environment, based on networked PCs, has for the first time given an opportunity for professionals without extensive computer backgrounds to implement and maintain effective information systems. Both libraries and social service organizations have benefited from this migration, particularly in smaller settings in which the cost of providing large computers and a centralized computing staff would never be feasible. The adoption of a distributed network environment and rapid growth of competing Internet service providers meant that individuals and small organizations could "rent" space on a network server and thereby provide access to their digital resource databases with little technical expertise and at very low cost. The cost and expertise required maintaining a Web page has become well within the capability of most small I&R agencies.

An important component of this process has been the accompanying education of the public for both understanding and using these technologies. Simply put, there is a considerable amount of expertise distributed throughout the public who accepts digital technologies and is able to use them. Testimony for the existence of this expertise is demonstrated in an oblique manner by the large and growing number of services and products that now advertise their e-mail and Web addresses to consumers. Clearly a critical mass of computer and network users exists to make such marketing efforts worthwhile. In the late 1980s, only a few thousand people in the United States, mostly employees of educational or research institutions, had e-mail addresses. Indeed, there was little awareness among the public and most professional workers of the nature of e-mail and data communications networks. Today millions of households send and receive electronic mail every day as a matter of course. Much of this e-mail is not confined to text but can include graphics, video and sound. Moreover, but an increasing number of individuals now have their own Web pages available for the world to scrutinize. It is not uncommon for new graduates of colleges and universities to refer prospective employers to their Web pages rather than mail paper resumes, because the Web page can add dimensions to a resume not possible in the paper product. The networked computer is rapidly becoming a major vehicle for social as well as for professional communication and interaction.

The I&R literature reflects the immense spread of computer technologies throughout the workplace during the 1990s. As early as 1990, an entire issue of the AIRS Journal was devoted to computerization of I&R activities (AIRS, 1990). I&R agencies were introducing automation and their staff had to grapple with problems of system selection and evaluation. Manikowski (1990) gave advice on how to choose an automated referral system and how to make automation decisions (Manikowski, 1990). Manikowski discussed all aspects of automating the resource file, including advantages and disadvantages of doing so. Pagano (1990) reported on a project by the Coalition to Prevent Substance Abuse and Suicide, Inc. for an online inventory of local substance abuse and mental health treatment and prevention agencies. The system included e-mail access for I&R professionals. There was also a recognition that automation coupled with network connectivity could create systems that spanned wide geographic areas. MacFadden, Carson, and Jackman describe the development of an automated network of information and referral services, an initiative of the Association of Community Information Centres in Ontario, Canada, to establish a major automated network of I&R services known as Online Ontario. The authors reported increases in efficiency among I&R centers due to the cooperation and sharing that the network made possible. The development of this network created a de facto standard for I&R services in that area. Concurrently, Maas (1990) advocated the sharing of jointly financed databases to provide a level of service that individual agencies on their own could not provide.

The 1990s also introduced a strong interest in developing intelligent computer systems—computer programs that embodied the knowledge of a human expert. The rationale for this effort was that human expertise was a scarce resource and that programming computer systems with intelligence might be an answer to this scarcity. The interest in expert systems was, to some extent, reflected in the I&R literature. Pittman & Kelly (1990) describe a prototype expert system for extracting I&R information from a resource file in response to queries. In the 1984 AIRS directory, approximately 90% of the reporting agencies indicated that they operate manual I&R systems. Of the agencies that reported the utilization of some type of automation, 19% reported that their resource files were computerized. The rest were using computers, presumably for administrative tasks. Indeed, Graves (1985) argued that computers in I&R agencies should be used in fiscal areas for managing and obtaining funds; determining client needs, and reevaluating areas for planning and organizing.

In a nationwide survey of library-based I&R services conducted by Childers in 1981, only 7% of the libraries reported use of computer equipment for their I&R resource files (Childers, 1984). The picture has changed dramatically since then. A national survey conducted by Levinson & Liebscher on a sample of 312 I&R agencies showed that 90% of I&R agencies now automated their resource files. Some caution must be used when interpreting these statistics since the I&R agencies surveyed tended to be larger agencies found in the AIRS directory. However, that was also the case in 1984 and so a strong trend toward computerization is evident. The incorporation of computers in I&R agencies spawned a great deal of "how-to" advice in journals and newsletters. One of the earliest such pieces appeared in the AIRS Newsletter on how to select the best system for an I&R agency (Provance, 1985). Schatt (1985) discussed a hands-on approach to preparing the agency for computerization including training, reducing stress, and migrating from manual to digital, and concluded that a consultant was probably necessary in most agencies. By 1988, the AIRS Newsletter contained a regular column by Dick Manikowski entitled "User-Friendly" that provided advice on dealing with a host of computer-related problems.

The rapid adoption of computer systems in I&R agencies coincided also with the growing recognition that this technology could facilitate the sharing of resources over computer networks. Steps were taken throughout the country to use computer networks for resource sharing. Woods (1996) outlined the planning process to put in place a digitally based community I&R network for the greater Rochester, New York, area. The major goals of the planners was to build a system that had a single, coordinated information system with unduplicated data; many points of access to accommodate varied customer and service provider needs; tighter information sharing among service providers to smooth transitions for customers; and the ability to transfer voice, data, and video via a telecommunications network.

Some I&R agencies, led by libraries who offered I&R services, explored the potential of the community free-nets that were springing up in cities throughout the country. Free-nets are electronic community bulletin board systems that can be accessed by community residents and that list information of interest to local residents. One of the earliest and best-known community free-nets is the Cleveland Free-net. Although a growing body of information is becoming available through access to online resources, there are still I&R providers who are not comfortable with giving clients direct access to this information. Assuming a public library perspective, Manikowski (1995) discusses points to consider before mounting electronic databases for direct patron access.

211 UNIVERSAL TELEPHONE ACCESS TO SERVICES—THE 2000'S

An information technology of long-standing and now ubiquitous in U.S. households is the telephone. In 1998 there were 63 telephones for every 100 Americans with an overall household penetration of almost 95%. Although access to telephones is lower among some minority groups such as African-Americans and Hispanics (approximately 70% of households) it is nevertheless the most available of the interactive information technologies (only radio penetration is higher with 205 radios per 100 population, but to date radio is not an interactive medium). I&R agencies have recognized the ubiquity of the telephone. An important component of first contact with I&R service providers has always been the telephone. As discussed in chapters 1 and 2, the continued fractionalization of I&R human services has created immense difficulties for citizens not only for finding appropriate services but also for finding appropriate I&R agencies. In effect the 1990s saw a growing interest among I&R service providers for centralized telephone access points.

By mid-2000, the Federal Communications Commission (FCC) granted the approval of the dialing code, 211 (or 2-1-1), for community information and referral nationwide. This approval has opened up a new chapter in the history of I&R and information technology, thereby providing universal access to new routes to helping services on all levels. Trained I&R specialists offer help over the telephone by linking 211 callers with needed information and services. Data were submitted to the FCC indicating that

211 provides a national safety network for persons in need that are *not* served by 911, 311, 800, or 888 numbers. The 311 telephone service was designed to reduce the number of nonemergency calls to 911 by providing access to nonemergency police centers. Hence, I&R specialists handling 211 calls can afford the time and attention to offer alternatives to callers that do not require emergency services. As shown in Figure 3.1, 211 is responsive to requests for information on human services and can also refer callers to other N11 numbers, as needed.

It is important to recognize the interest that the Atlanta and Connecticut 211 programs have generated in other states in implementing the 211 exchange. By mid-2000, members of the National Collaborative for 211 numbered 30 partnering organizations that committed themselves to the implementation of 211. Following the lead of United Way in Atlanta, a campaign to include a 211 number in all communities that connects "citizens with problems" with appropriate I&R agencies was conducted. The 211 service in Atlanta provides a free telephone help line 24 hours a day, 7 days a week and is supported by a database of more than 800 I&R agencies and direct callers to needed services. It is estimated that I&R organizations across the United States answer more than 50 million calls each year.

Other states and local communities are engaged in serious discussions with plans to adopt 211 as an established community service. In Texas, for example, the state Senate studied the possibility of 211 services that would allow parents, police, teachers, and others to quickly access information about gang intervention, counseling, and assistance programs (IR Networker, Oct. 1998). On May 28, 1998, AIRS and five other partner organizations filed a petition with the FCC requesting that the 211 dialing code be set aside as a national phone number for access to community resources, much as 911 is reserved for emergencies. On July 21, 2000 the FCC granted the abbreviated dialing code, 211, for community information and referral nationwide.

In discussing options for implementing state-of-the art telephone technology, Lori Warrens, executive director of United Way 211 in Atlanta, noted that the single toll-free telephone to reach I&R services not only changed the metro area perception of I&R, but has also been a catalyst for upgrading the I&R center telephone system in ways that were unimaginable heretofore (Warrens, 1999). It is logical that this telephone revolution will generate increased need for professional training and supervision in the helping process via telephone. Increased demands for knowledge of telephone communication and technology will be imperative. It is expected

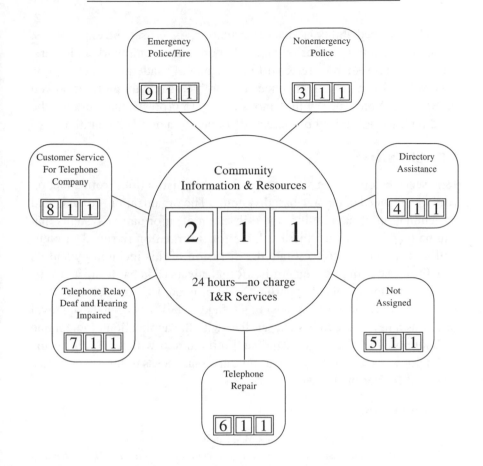

Figure 3.1 Identification of the national 211 telephone system and other N11 services.*

* 111—not applicable.
Source: "AIRS Creating a 211 Service." *211 Partners.* April 28, 1999, pp. 6–7.

that it will take time to create a nationwide 211 network. I&R telephone systems are currently in the process of being upgraded and are involved in basic telephone technology, including available options. I&R staff are becoming far more informed on what telephone systems to consider as they recognize the need to gain required skills in telephone assistance to callers.

Rapid advances in wireless technologies have made it possible for the public to communicate by voice, phone and video, and to connect to a large number of databases through small, handheld devices from anywhere in the world. These same technologies will soon provide professionals with a much-enhanced ability to share information, expertise, and experiences. Future barriers to cooperation and collaboration among workers in various professions such as I&R will not be one of inadequate technology. That will exist in great abundance. The problems remaining to be solved are far more concerned with demonstrating, to professional workers, the need for and desirability of increased cooperation and collaboration.

CONCLUSIONS

I&R services operate at varying levels of sophistication, from shoebox files to advanced computer-based systems. The organization, storage, and dissemination of data require the utilization of information systems that can be readily accessed and available for information retrieval. A compelling challenge is to facilitate the diffusion of this technology and its benefits to the entire I&R enterprise. Rapid advances in hardware and software offer unprecedented opportunities to promote I&R operational effectiveness. A crowning achievement in the field of I&R has been the approval of 211 as a new route to human services with the application of telephone technology. The challenge of the new millennium will be to utilize this technology in the interest of securing universal access to human services, analyzed further in chapter 4.

REFERENCES

AIRS *Newsletter*. (1983, March–June). Brief notes.

AIRS. (1990). Special issue on automation. *Information & Referral: The Journal of the Alliance of Information and Referral Systems, 12* (1–2), 1–55.

Bellamy, D. E., & Forgie, D. J. (1984). Impact of advanced technology on I&R in a Canadian provincial context. In R. W. Levinson, & K. Haynes (Eds.), *Accessing human services: International perspectives* (pp. 199–215). Beverly Hills, CA: Sage.

Childers, T. (1984). *Information and referral. Public libraries.* Norwood, NJ: Ablex.

Ferguson, T. (1996). *Health online: How to find health information, support group, and self-help communities in cyberspace.* New York: Addison Wesley.

Garrett, W. (1984). Technological advances in I&R: An American report. In R. W. Levinson, & K. S. Haynes (Eds.), *Accessing human services: International perspectives* (pp. 171–198). Beverly Hills, CA: Sage.

Geiss, G. R., & Viswanathan, N. (1986). *The human edge: Information technology and helping people.* New York: The Haworth Press.

Graves, A. S. (1985). No longer a question of "if," but "when." *AIRS Newsletter, 13* (4), 1.

Haynes, K. S., & Sallee, A. L. (1979). Information and referral: A database for social planners. *Information and Referral: The Journal of the Alliance of Information and Referral Systems, 1* (1), 51–63.

Levinson, R. W. (1988). *Information and referral networks: Doorways to human services.* New York: Springer Publishing.

Maas, N. L. (1990). The challenge of building shared I&R databases. *Information and Referral: The Journal of the Alliance of Information and Referral Systems, 12* (1–2), 52–55.

Manikowski, D. (1995). Making referral file automation decisions. *Information and Referral: The Journal of the Alliance of Information and Referral Systems, 17,* 85–107.

McFadden, R. J., Carson, D., & Jackman, M. (1990). Electronic Community: Developing an automated network of information and referral services. *Information and Referral: The Journal of the Alliance of Information and Referral Systems, 12* (1–2), 32–51.

Pagano, S. V. (1990). CPSAS, In./Iona College ACHRIS@ program. *Information and Referral: The Journal of the Alliance of Information and Referral Systems, 12* (1–2), 28–31.

Pittman, S. A., & Kelly, M. J. (1990). ILRA: A knowledge-based system link to an electronic resource file. *Information and Referral: The Journal of the Alliance of Information and Referral Systems, 12* (1–2), 16–27.

Provance, J. L. (1985). Choosing a system: Invest time before money. *AIRS Newsletter, 13* (5), 6.

Puryear, D. (1982). Early I&R programs in libraries. *Information and Referral: The Journal of the Alliance of Information and Referral Systems, 4* (2), 16–20.

Schatt, L. (1985). The day the computer arrives. *AIRS Newsletter, 13* (6), 1.

Sherman, B. (1986). *Information and Referral: The Journal of the Alliance Information and Referral Systems, 8* (2), 000–000.

Sullivan, R. J. (1979). Computerized information and referral: An introduction. *Information and Referral: The Journal of the Alliance of Information and Referral Systems, 1* (3), 13–24.

Vanderheiden, G. C. (1989). Development of an ultra-user friendly, disseminable database system for information and referral. *Information and Referral: The Journal of the Alliance of Information and Referral Systems, 11* (1–2), 49–65.

Wimberley, E. T., Blazyk, S., Crawford, C., & Hokanson, J. (1987). Improving care coordination for geriatric patients: Computer-assisted case management. *Information and Referral: The Journal of the Alliance of Information and Referral Systems, 9* (1), 1–13.

Woods, D. (1996). The I&R heart of community-wide networks: HelpNet, a model under construction. *Information and Referral: The Journal of the Alliance of Information and Referral Systems, 18,* 7–20.

PART II

Provision of I&R Services in a Digital Age

CHAPTER 4

The Basics of I&R Service Delivery

*In order for the promise of universal service to become a reality,
people need to be able to obtain the information they require in a
way that is meaningful to them, regardless of their technological
sophistication, first language, income or other factors.*
Georgia Sales, 1995

The multifaceted role of I&R within the vast array of human services essentially performs a linkage function by "bringing people and services together." The broad term of "human services" is an all-inclusive term for the totality of organized programs that promote the health and social welfare of all persons, groups, and communities. Although social services and health services tend to be regarded as independent service systems, the application of Information and Referral services bridges both service systems and intersects in a wide variety of service patterns.

THE ROLE OF I&R WITHIN THE HUMAN SERVICES

Since the early 1960s, organized I&R services have developed concurrently within three major categories of human services: comprehensive, specialized, and crisis-disaster services. As discussed in chapter 1 (Figure 1.1), human services are broadly categorized as comprehensive or universal services (social utilities). A second category is defined as personal services (social cases) that respond to specific needs and problems of individuals and families. A third category of services to which I&R is uniquely responsive is disaster services, which includes crises services that occur as both public and personal concerns and that may present serious and often life-threatening conditions. Because of the capability of I&R to respond not only to personal emergencies but also to public catastrophes with needed information and referrals to helping sources, I&R has gained recognition as a highly responsive service that is capable of connecting persons with needed resources under crisis and disaster conditions.

As noted in Table 4.1 on Categories of Human Services, which are reported in the AIRS 1995–1996 directory, more than half of the reported agencies are involved in generic or comprehensive services. Thus, the universal role of I&R impacts on all phases of the life span in promoting quality of life, such as public health, housing, recreation, public education, and public safety programs. As many as 109 agencies reported services to the aging, which constitute the highest number of "life cycle I&R programs."

A second category of services focuses more specifically on individuals, families, and specific groups who require information and assistance with their problems and concerns such as personal health conditions, mental illness, and disability. The AIRS directory lists 245 specialized agencies, which represent 35% of the total number of agencies. Beginning with the late 1960s and continuing through successive decades, consumer demands, spurred by special interest groups, highlighted the need for specialized services for specific target groups. Among the specialized services that

TABLE 4.1 Categories of Human Services

I	**79.3%**	Comprehensive Services—*Social Utilities*		**557**
		Generic Services	77.6%	432
		Life Cycle Services	22.4%	125
		Aging 109		
		Children/Youth 12		
		Women 4		
II	**17.1%**	Specialized Services—*Social Cases*		**120**
		Military	67.5%	81
		Disability	13.3%	16
		Health Related	11.7%	14
		Sectarian—Ethnic Related	4.2%	5
		Drug/Alcohol	2.5%	3
		Literacy	0.8%	1
III	**3.6%**	Disaster/Crisis		**25**
		Disaster	60.0%	15
		Crisis	40.0%	10
	100%	**TOTAL**		**702**

Source: Directory of Information and Referral Systems. *Alliance of Information and Referral Systems, Inc. and United Way of America* (1995–1996). Joliet, IL: Author.

received funding have been I&R programs for people who are chronically ill, disabled, or disenfranchised, as well for the new immigrant groups.

Despite the dramatic advances in the world of medicine, and not withstanding the expending volume of social services, access to health care continues to be a serious problem. The list of blockages to health services has become even more extended due to financial barriers, maldistribution of service locations, inconvenient hours, and shifting health costs are taken into account. According to Titmuss (1968), "the uniquely disadvantaged health consumer" is often in no position to shop around in a competitive marketplace for health-related services. Furthermore, health problems are often unpredictable, sometimes catastrophic, and may in fact suggest life-and-death implications. The symbiotic term, "health and welfare" often used synonymously and interchangeably, suggests absolute interdependence of these two concepts. The introduction of Medicare in the mid-1960s and Health Maintenance Organizations in the 1980s has brought a host of new benefits. To qualify for the various Medicare options and other health plans that have evolved since the 1980s, information and referral services can make a great difference. I&R has demonstrated the capacity to clarify and to assist consumers in arriving at informed choices for health care.

The third category of human services to which I&R is responsive involves personal and public emergencies that deal with crises and catastrophic conditions. The AIRS directory (1995–1996) lists 25 agencies that respond to emergency situations which include both comprehensive and specialized I&R agencies. Because of the unique capabilities of I&R to respond to all kinds of crisis situations, these emergency services constitute a third category of human services. Historically, the emergency conditions of World War II brought about the development of Citizens Advice Bureaus in the United Kingdom. In the United States, veterans' postwar needs generated the emergency programs of Veterans Information Centers. As reported in the historical development of I&R (chap. 2), crisis information centers for drug and alcohol addiction and suicide prevention programs were among the earliest of reported I&R programs in the Bloksberg survey (Bloksberg & Caso, 1967). To cover crisis calls that are received after regular office hours, growing numbers of social agencies arrange to transfer callers to I&R services that operate beyond the usual office hours.

Agencies also operate their own hot lines, a telephone service that may also be staffed by I&R volunteers who are trained to respond to emergencies.

Peer-group members, who may have special understanding and empathy with the callers, may compose crises line staff. The growing numbers of hot lines indicate the pressing need of people in crises or perceived crisis situations to obtain information and reach help without undue delay, as reported by Laudisio (1993) in her description of Hurricane Andrew's impact on I&R. A hot-line request may entail a single contact or more extensive contacts between the client and the I&R agent. In either case, hot lines rely on effective working relationships with other human service organizations to expedite referrals for emergency conditions (Roberts, 1995). I&R agencies often operate one or more hot-line services in addition to their regular service program, such as the Vancouver Information Service, which succeeded, with the aid of government contracts, to operate both a domestic violence hot line and a substance abuse hot line—both of which are available to all the residents of British Columbia.

I&R services have increasingly become active in disaster situations since the decade of the 1990s. The 1993 special edition of the AIRS journal reported on the involvement of selected AIRS agencies during several disasters, including hurricanes, volcanic eruptions, and earthquakes. Local I&R programs played a critical role in coordinating information following the aftermath of Hurricane Hugo in Charlotte, North Carolina (Nance, 1993); the earthquake and fires in the bay area of San Francisco (Wallrich, 1998); the hurricanes in Florida, Louisiana, and Hawaii (Dray, Salmers, & Larsen, 1993); and the riots, fires, and earthquakes in Los Angeles (Wallrich, 1993). I&R staff from Info Line of Los Angeles were still providing services in Appalachian Centers more than a year after the Northridge quake that struck in 1994. United Way of Charlotte, North Carolina, and the Switchboard of Miami also reported on their role in recovery from Hurricane Andrew described as "the storm of the century."

Experience in disaster situations has indicated that "few events stretch human capacity and challenge individuals and communities to adapt to rapidly changing environmental conditions like a major disaster" (Webster, 1995). The results may be traumatic disruptions to normal living patterns and serious economic losses as well as lack of provisions for human care. In discussing the role of Switchboard of Miami, the need for preparedness was recognized as crucially important (Laudisio, 1993). I&R's role involved negotiating agreements with the Federal Emergency Management Association, the Red Cross, and the Voluntary Organizations Active in a Disaster. These organizational networks were vital in service delivery for immediate assistance and for future planning of optimum survival under disaster conditions. One of the major contributions to the recovery efforts following disaster conditions has been the utilization of the resource files and service directories maintained by I&R agencies. An unanticipated finding that resulted from involvement in the aftermath of the hurricane in Dade County (Laudisio, 1993) was the realization that serious gaps in existing service programs did not permit effective and efficient emergency responses.

Not all disasters are a result of natural catastrophes. Info Line of California detailed their activities during the civil disturbances following the verdict in the first Rodney King beating trial in greater Los Angeles (Wallrich, 1993). The Memphis library-based I&R service known as LINC (Gandy, 1993), reported on the disruptive impact of the Operation Desert Watch in their community. Among the items discussed were relationships with other organizations, community-wide volunteer involvement, and special roles for referring agencies during times of disaster.

As comprehensive, specialized, and emergency I&R services have continued to develop concurrently, two trends have become evident. Although I&R services often begin as specialized services for target populations, such as the handicapped and battered women, requests for general information may be required. On the other hand, as general I&R services expand to include larger groups of users, the need for specialized information may be apparent. If the specialized service is not available within the agency's range of services, appropriate referrals are either sought from other organizations, or the agency itself may develop specialized services. A case in point is the increased specialization within the British Citizens Advice Bureau (CAB) programs, which are basically local public information agencies staffed by more than 90% volunteers. However, since the early 1980s it became apparent that paid specialists were needed to respond to marital and family counseling, welfare benefits, and housing and consumer affairs (NACAB, 2000).

THE BASICS OF I&R OPERATIONS

MODES OF ENTRY

The client's entry to I&R services varies, depending on whether the initial request is made by telephone, by mail, by walk-in, or by e-mail. In the United States, the telephone is the most prevalent mode of access to I&R

services for inquirers. Telephone communications have been enhanced through toll-free 800 numbers, tie-lines, and various technical capabilities such as call-waiting, call-forwarding, and three-way calling, which link the caller to the service provider via the referral agent. A significant breakthrough in direct phone access has been the introduction of the 24-hour cost-free 211 local phone service, which was approved by the Federal Communication Commission on July 21, 2000.

Another mode of entry is the I&R walk-in service, which is usually conducted at convenient locations such as town halls, public libraries, transit centers, or at store-front service centers. Open-door services are exceedingly helpful when a face-to-face meeting is required for practical assistance in completing formal applications, or when a more detailed report or a more accurate assessment is needed to arrive at a service plan. Since walk-in services require available staff who are prepared to respond directly to client inquiries, it is important to judiciously assess the demand and volume of services that can possibly be handled by I&R service staff, otherwise the demand may exceed the volume of cases that the I&R agency can accommodate. User-operated kiosks are increasingly being used by the public as convenient sources for information.

A nationwide survey of local public libraries conducted by Levinson and Liebscher in 1996–1997 reported a high percentage of I&R walk-ins compared with phone requests. However, the responding librarians indicated that there is a trend for an increase in I&R telephone inquiries. A limited but generally unreported number of requests are received by mail. One possible reason for mail inquiries may be the person's lack of a telephone. Another likelihood is that inquirers may be reluctant to ask for help or to discuss problems by telephone because of embarrassment, stigma, or difficulties in articulation or language problems. The volume of written inquiries is generally quite limited. If the request for a service requires referral to another agency, the client's permission must be obtained before sending a copy of the original letter to the referred agency. These operational procedures aim to safeguard confidentiality, which governs all aspects of I&R services (Jacobson, 1994).

The expanding application of e-mail and searches on the Internet serve as prompt and efficient means to make a personal connection to an I&R resource. As technology has become more available to larger groups of users, the dramatic increase in the volume of inquiries by e-mail has significantly expanded. It is clearly indicated that the e-mail mode of service inquiry will continue to expand, and the availability of a vast range of helping services can be sought by "surfing the Internet." As noted previously, a highly significant development in access to services has been the approval of the 211 universal telephone services, which will continue to expand as I&R agencies institute their own 211 telephone systems.

CLIENT-CENTERED I&R SERVICE COMPONENTS

For purposes of analysis and comprehensiveness, the components of I&R-helping services are divided into two major categories: *client-centered services* to I&R consumers, and *agency-centered services* that focus on organizational operations that deal with policy, planning, outreach, administration, and research. Rather than regarding I&R as a series of discrete service modules, I&R practice indicates that the elements or components of an I&R program are functionally interrelated, operate interactively, and tend to be perceived as a continuum. The continuum may range from assistance with information only to advising and counseling. The extent of information given may depend upon the nature of the specific inquiry and the level at which the information can be appropriately shared with the inquirer. Given the complexity and multiplicity of human problems, what may initially appear as a request for simple information may in fact be a complex situation that will require referral to another appropriate resource or multiple resources.

TABLE 4.2 Continua of I&R Specialist Intervention in Direct I&R Services to Clientele

Direct I&R Services	Less Intervention ⟶ More Intervention		
Basic I&R Components	Information ⟶ Assistance	Referral	⟶ Follow-up
Support Services	Translation ⟶ Services	Transportation	⟶ Escort Services
Case Advocacy	Initiation of ⟶ Case by Specialist	Case Defense	⟶ Case Referral to Legal Services if Indicated
Interpersonal Relationships with Client	Inform ⟶	Advise	⟶ Counsel

As illustrated in Table 4.2, direct I&R services are viewed as continua of functional components that range from "less intervention" to "more intervention" by the service provider. Information assistance, referral, and follow-up are viewed as the basic components. These tasks relate to the continuum of interpersonal relations that may range from information only (steering) to advice and counseling. If language communication is a problem, translation services may be made available. To ensure client travel to a given destination, transportation and possibly personal escort services may be provided.

Information Provision

The basic functions of I&R involve assisting with needed information, providing referrals, and conducting follow-up. The largest volume of requests for I&R services is primarily in the area of "I" (information) rather than "R" (referral) on the continuum of I&R service delivery. Information assistance may be offered in response to simple and straightforward inquiries such as how to get a copy of a birth certificate or what veterans benefits are available to help finance graduate studies. Going beyond simple information inquiries, information may be requested for more complex matters dealing with personal problem that are concerned with entitlements, benefits, or legal provision, as noted in the following situations:

1. "Can my mother-in-law be committed to a mental institution under nonvoluntary conditions?"
2. "I have been fired twice within the past 6 months; how do I apply for unemployment compensation?"
3. "In buying a home, am I entitled to an exemption as a veteran?"

To respond to these inquiries, background information about the inquirer is necessary to determine entitlements or potential eligibility. Referral of the consumer to an appropriate service may require minimal or, as indicated, far more extensive intervention. What is described as a simple referral may be handled by the "steering process," which involves providing sufficient information to enable the inquirer to follow through independently. A complex referral may, however, require more active intervention by the provider, such as making an appointment for the client with a staff member at another agency, writing a letter, or actually representing the client, if necessary. What may initially appear to be a simple referral may, in fact, turn out to be a far more complex situation. For example, a request for the address of a family planning agency may involve a simple referral to a public health clinic or to the office of a Planned Parenthood agency. However, when the same inquiry is presented with the additional information that "I think I'm pregnant and my parents must not know," the referral process is no longer simple.

How a simple request can mount into a complex problem is further illustrated by the following situation:

An inquirer may ask for information on a local pharmacy for the purchase of medication at a discount rate. Further discussion may reveal that the caller is the mother of a 7-year-old child and that her husband who is currently unemployed has incurred heavy debts to the extent that he is unable to meet the family's present living expenses. The care of two younger children, aged 2 and 5, has ruled out the possibility of the mother's working. In addition to being overwhelmed with the child's diagnosis as epileptic, the mother states that she is particularly agitated by her husband's resentment that she did not tell him prior to their marriage that her maternal grandfather had epilepsy.

The complexity of this case may call for multiple referrals, repeated contacts with the inquirer, additional contacts with other members of the family, and a variety of referrals to relevant and appropriate agencies. The situation may demand more than simple information assistance and referral. For the child with epilepsy, the I&R agent may be forced to probe for underlying problems in the seemingly simple request for discount drugs. What did the I&R worker regard as the primary problem? Was it the child's epilepsy, the husband's unemployment, or the wife's overwhelming efforts to handle family pressures? The outcome of this case ultimately will depend upon the I&R agent's delineation of the problem and the handling of referrals with the available and appropriate agencies. To meet some of the family's needs, referrals may involve not only discount drug suppliers, but also the child's local school, contact with the unemployment office, job-training programs for the father, and referral to a family service agency or a mental health center, or other counseling services. Rather than engaging in multiple referrals, it is conceivable that the complex family problems may be most effectively and efficiently handled by a single referral to a local chapter of the Epilepsy Foundation of America, if available.

Referral and Follow-Up

Referral and follow-up are logically regarded as a dual process based on the assumption that a referral implies some measure of follow-up. However, in practice, universal follow-up on all inquiries usually occurs only under special circumstances, such as a requirement for a particular project or a special study within a limited period of time or for purposes of quality control or program evaluation. Follow-up may also be conducted on a priority basis, a procedure followed by various I&R agencies in New York City that prioritize requests for fuel allowances for older persons during severe cold weather in the winter.

The main purpose of follow-up is to determine whether the service has been delivered and whether the outcome is satisfactory. At the time of the initial client contact, follow-up procedures should be explained by the service provider, clearly indicating that it is carried out only with the user's consent, except under emergency or other unusual circumstance. To help guide staff with referral procedures, it is advisable that agency policies on current referral procedures be clearly spelled out in a set of instructions or a published policy manual. Why do some referrals fail or remain pending? Perhaps the information was insufficient, unclear, or inappropriate. If misinformation has been inadvertently given, efforts should be made to rectify the error promptly and enter the corrected information into the agency resource files. Ideally, both the client and the referred agency are contacted in a follow-up plan. The more common practice is to contact the client, however, since agency follow-up may entail issues of organizational competition or turf. A more subtle reason is that follow-up may imply an evaluative judgment on the performance of the referred agency by the referring I&R service.

In the final analysis, the degree of follow-up depends upon the gravity and complexity of the situation, the policy of the I&R organization, and the judgment of the I&R agent. It also depends upon the availability of resources, the limitations of staff time, and the costs involved. A critical issue in follow-up is confidentiality, because a case referral usually requires identification of the caller by the referring agency (Kitkowski, 2000; Jacobson, 1994).

Support Services

To carry out a responsible service, it may be necessary to provide support services, depending upon service needs. Because of the increased numbers of ethnic groups who have arrived in the United States since the 1970s, I&R agencies are finding that translation services are essential. Growing numbers of I&R agencies are therefore using bilingual volunteers or hiring staff with multilingual capabilities. Many bilingual directories are also made available for the convenience of the non–English speaking client and thereby available for direct use by the client. As many as 130 languages are used for I&R services in the Community Information Toronto agency. Translator services are also available in ethnic-specific I&R agencies such as the Service Directory for Chinatown in New York City. When travel to needed services is a problem for the client, I&R agencies may provide their own transportation or arrange for transportation with an outside agency. Escort services may also be provided by I&R staff members to give support, supply needed information, or negotiate with another service system on behalf of the client.

Case Advocacy

In case advocacy, the assumption is that the person in need of services is unable to engage in self-advocacy. Under these conditions, case advocacy is conducted to remedy or ameliorate a specific problem or a given situation for an individual or family (Blakely, 1991). When the client is unable to deal with the barriers to services, or in situations where the client has been mistreated or inadequately dealt with, case advocacy may be the necessary course of action to make complaint or redress a grievance. In dealing with problems that involve organizational neglect or ineptitude in the delivery of client services, the case advocate may find it necessary to resort to higher levels of supervisory or administrative personnel. In addition, the case advocate may have to institute an appeal process or refer the client to a professional lawyer if further litigation is involved. To delineate professional roles that relate to the possible unauthorized practice of law, Kahn drew a helpful distinction between "legal assistance," which can appropriately be supplied by an I&R specialist agent, and "legal services," for which a client requires a referral to a professional attorney (Kahn, 1966).

Interpersonal Relationships

The intensity and duration of the interpersonal aspects of the I&R process tend to vary with the nature of the problem and the level of the working relationship with the client. In the process of I&R counseling, the first step is usually to provide a necessary assessment of the inquirer's presenting problem and to clarify the inquirer's circumstances. A second step may require suggesting a course of action, thereby exerting a stronger degree of intervention by the provider. Based upon a delineation of the problem situation, the I&R specialist may, upon a review of alternatives with the client, arrive at a plan for action or refer the client to an appropriate outside agency. If in-depth counseling or therapy is indicated, a referral to an agency may be appropriate. Operationally, the extent and intensity of counscling depend upon the nature of the inquiry, the capacity of the client's follow-through, and the service program of the particular I&R agency.

In the absence of a unitary model of the I&R interview process, Maas suggested "three models to remember" represented by Long (1921), Caplan (1964) and Besser (1983)." Maas cited Long's formulation of "interviewing and information giving" relevant to the interviewing process. As a psychologist, Long detailed the interviewing process with sensitivity to the dual relationship between the interviewer and the interviewee, noting that "I&R is an access point and an entryway to a large and complicated service network that is designed to help people in its own cumbersome way" (Interstudy, 1971). A second model cited by Maas is the crisis intervention model based on Gerald Caplan's (1964) seminal work on preventive psychiatry. With a focus on self-help, Maas also recommended a third approach to the interview process by applying active listening skills, as suggested in the *How to Hot Line Manual* by Besser (1983). These models represent a rich heritage of guiding principles for the challenging and sensitive process involved in conducting an I&R interview. Maas suggested that each of these models was worthy of consideration and emphasized the skills in active listening as a quick and efficient way to develop rapport in any situation. According to Maas, active listening skills can prove helpful in becoming more sensitive, empathetic, and objective listeners.

AGENCY-CENTERED I&R SERVICES COMPONENTS

In addition to the direct services, I&R programs also include a broad array of indirect services, including planning, policy advocacy, outreach, and publicity. So vital are these indirect services to quality I&R practice that the effectiveness of I&R services clearly depends upon the sound implementation and effective management of the following agency-centered I&R services.

Planning & Research

Optimal utilization of I&R data for planning purposes requires documented data that are valid and applicable to sufficiently large numbers of clientele to support the reliability of the reported data. To overcome possible resistance to documentation, involvement of I&R staffing in the early phases of data selection and explanation of why and how the data will be used are necessary. The AIRS/INFO LINE Taxonomy provides a common language for identification of terminology and thereby provides an opportunity for consistent reporting of services. To arrive at clear instructions for documentation, a testing period can be helpful to revise and modify data forms as indicated. In considering the extent to which I&R data may be used for social planning purposes, Long observed rather soberly that social planning is essentially a political process in which decisions are often arrived at to accommodate political pressures, irrespective of the nature of the data findings (Long, 1973). Nevertheless, given the need for empirical data, I&R programs can provide databases for rational decision making and budgetary allocations in social planning. However, the validity of the data reported will depend upon whether the I&R services meet acceptable standards and criteria (Standards, 2000).

Policy Advocacy

Unlike case advocacy, which focuses on the individual client, policy or class advocacy is generally concerned with the experience of aggregates of consumers in I&R programs. The policy advocate may be involved in social action, legislative changes, or community education, depending on the area of concern. To illustrate, an annual report of an I&R agency noted that more calls were received requesting transportation services for older persons than were recorded for any other single category of consumer requests during a given year. Upon staff review and approval from the executive board and other appropriate levels of agency administration, the I&R agency considered one of several alternative courses of action in arriving at a policy decision to meet transportation needs: A policy decision may be made that the I&R agency will operate its own minibus in a given area, provided that local fraternal and civic organizations will contribute to the purchase of a bus. Or the policy advocate may encourage concerned citizens to write to legislators requesting funds for a transportation plan that will be jointly supported by a grant from the state office on the aging and contributory funds from the local county. Another strategy may involve a series of radio announcements or TV shorts that will dramatize the plight of older people, who, because of lack of adequate transportation as documented in I&R case records, do not have the means to reach available services. An even more effective tactic might be the formation of groups of older citizens known to the I&R agency who will campaign for transportation services by attending legislative sessions and conducting town hall meetings. Based on systematically reported data, the I&R agency may consider any of the above options that could lead to changes in service provision.

Outreach & Publicity

An I&R service is usually activated by a client request with the I&R provider as responder or reactor. However, the I&R provider can also assume the role of an initiator by reaching out to target groups to recruit potential clientele. Since the extent to which an I&R service is utilized depends upon the community's awareness of the service, a vigorous public relations program should be conducted to reach the uninformed and uninvolved, but potentially interested, consumer. Outreach may involve the operation of mobile I&R services in remote rural areas or for hard-to-reach older populations in a suburban area or inner-city region. Systematic outreach may require a time-phased plan for canvassing potential consumers to inform them of the availability of I&R services. Emergency outreach programs may also be conducted by I&R agencies to alert the community to a common concern, a pending disaster, or environmental problems such as air pollution or lead poisoning. A public education program or possibly a survey may be conducted to inform the community about the high incidence of reported substance abuse or the problems of unemployed youth as reflected in I&R service requests. Distribution of specialized directories is also effective for outreach and publicity. Cueny (1990) reports that 20,000 free directories are distributed to older persons (The Survivor Guide) and 20,000 students receive the Youth Yellow Pages through the school system.

Canvassing local neighborhoods and engaging in publicity programs through public service announcements on radio and TV can be effective for this group as well. One of the consequences of outreach efforts is the development of new groups of I&R consumers. For example, librarians discovered that library-based I&R programs attract a totally new group of inquirers, over and beyond the traditional book-borrowing patrons.

THE RESOURCE DATABASE: TAXONOMY

Each I&R program or agency organizes its resource files to enable an I&R specialist to quickly and easily find the resource information appropriate to the client's needs. Files may be organized alphabetically by agency name, or by using a set of key words that describe an agency's services, or a standardized indexing system, which is known as a taxonomy. The value of using a taxonomy is twofold: First, agencies that share a common classification system can more easily share resource information. Second, a common classification method allows the I&R community to more effectively compare and analyze referral activity across agencies. The challenge of using a taxonomy is learning its "vocabulary" and appropriately applying it to each resource in the file.

The AIRS/INFO LINE Taxonomy is a classification system that allows organizations maintaining human-services databases to index and access community resources based on the services they provide and the target groups they serve. The Taxonomy provides a framework for a common language for human services. It ensures that the field has common concepts, common terminology for naming services, and agreements regarding definitions for what a service involves. Not only does the Taxonomy allow users to identify appropriate resources for specific clients, it also supports the ability of users to collect and share statistical information. The Taxonomy provides a common ground for collaboration of services involving professionals from different disciplines, for organizations engaging in human services research, and for communities committed to the development of database cooperatives. The Taxonomy provides a common language for the human services and is being used by more than 400 I&R programs, libraries, crisis lines, and similar programs throughout North America to access information about organizations and their resource files.

The Taxonomy features a five-level hierarchical structure that contains 4,300 terms which are organized into 10 basic categories. Figure 4.1 provides a listing of the 10 basic categories. The sample from the Hierarchy (Figure 4.2) displays the logic and rationale of matching service categories within a hierarchy of social service terms.

In the service field of disaster services, a Taxonomy of Human Services

• Basic Subsistence	• Income Security
• Consumer Services	• Individual and Family Life
• Criminal Justice and Legal Services	• Mental Health Care and Counseling
• Education	• Organizational/Community Services
• Environmental Quality	• Target Groups
• Health Care	

Figure 4.1 Basic categories of the Taxonomy of Human Services.

Source: A Taxonomy of Human Services: A Conceptual Framework with Standardized Terminology and Definitions for the Field, 1994. Out of the Shadows, in AIRS 1995, Illinois: Joliet. Reprinted with permission.

was developed in 1998 by Georgia Sales, Burt Wallrich, and Bill Butler as part of the AIRS NERIN project (National Emergency Response Information Network) projects. This taxonomy contains terminology that can be used to index and access disaster-related services in both predisaster and postdisaster databases as described in the resource protocols component of the NERIN model. Predisaster databases contain information about organizations with disaster preparedness, mitigation, response, relief, and recovery responsibility, which can be available prior to the occurrence of the disaster. Familiarity with the disaster services section of the taxonomy should help in planning for the types of services that are needed to identify and to develop a timetable during a disaster (Sales, 1998).

There are two vital concerns regarding the taxonomy: (a) What are the inclusion/exclusion criteria in determining the scope of the resource file? and (b) What is the indexing process in maintaining the AIRS/INFO LINE taxonomy?

INCLUSIVE/EXCLUSIVE CRITERIA

In reply to the first question, agencies require guidelines that explicitly state what criteria qualify an agency for inclusion in the file and what conditions disqualify the agency (Manikowski, 2000). Clearly, there is a need to establish and publish guidelines. There is also a need for disclaimers of responsibility where appropriate. The guidelines for agency inclusion/exclusion criteria should be explicitly written and used consistently, not only on a case-by-case decision. Manikowski notes that inclusion of for-profit agencies are to be considered under specific conditions. Inclusion does not imply endorse-

---

Terms that appear in the Taxonomy of Human Services: A Conceptual Framework with Standardized Terminology and Definitions for the Field 1994.

BH Housing:
Programs that seek to meet the basic shelter needs of the community by providing temporary shelter for people who are in emergency situations, home improvements, housing location assistance, and a variety of housing alternatives. See also Homesteading Assistance.
   (FT-330), Landlord/Tenant assistants
   (FT-450), Leisure Accommodations
   (PL-450)

BH-180 Emergency Shelter:
Programs that provide a temporary place to stay for newcomers, travelers, people who are in crisis, or homeless individuals in the community.

BH-180.150   Crisis Shelter:
Programs that provide a temporary place to stay for people who are unable to return to their own homes due to sexual assault, domestic violence, or other problems. See also Disaster Shelter.
   (JR-150.150-19), Crisis Houses (RP-150.150)

BH-180.150-10 Battered Women's Shelter:
Programs that provide temporary emergency shelter for women who have experienced domestic violence, and for their children. Such facilities usually, in-house individual, group, and family counseling and a full range of secondary services related to domestic violence, including referral to appropriate resources.

Figure 4.2 Sample from the Hierarchy.

Source: Out of the Shadows. *AIRS,* 1994.

ment. A general rule of thumb is that for-profit agencies are included if non-profit agencies do not offer the specific service that is needed.

INDEXING THE TAXONOMY

In discussing the second question on indexing, the process entails accurate and consistent indexing. Customizing the taxonomy entails "striking a balance between what people want and need and what is feasible for the I&R program to maintain." Bruni's article on indexing serves as a guide for the process of indexing the taxonomy. Keeping the taxonomy current with new terms and references makes it a very useful tool. Selecting indexing terms from the taxonomy gives I&R providers the assurance that they are using the terminology and definitions that are recognized and endorsed by the I&R field. Thus, users achieve the dual objectives of a standard classification scheme while having the flexibility to index their individual agency files. A report on Connecticut's experience on "customizing" the taxonomy attests to the flexibility of adapting the taxonomy to meet the state's individual needs (Hogan).

AN "A" CHECKLIST: ATTRIBUTES OF AN I&R SERVICE

In the ongoing process of formulating acceptable standards and criteria for I&R practice, there appears to be a growing consensus on the various qualities that are considered essential for an acceptable I&R practice. The following is a suggested "A" checklist of ten essential attributes for I&R services.

Availability.

Is the I&R service universally available, unbiased, and nonpartisan? Are extended waiting periods avoided? Are services offered as purported? What measures must be considered for the installation and operation of the 211 telephone system?

Accessibility.

Can the service be conveniently reached? Are phone lines open for all callers? Is entry uncomplicated? Can the inquirer make direct contact with I&R staff or independently use database files? Is the database appropriately and adequately indexed to identify specific categories of services within the agency's taxonomy?

Appropriateness.

Does the I&R program meet the needs and preferences of the general population or specific target group it aims to serve? Are the referrals appropriate to suit the specific concerns of the client? What opportunities are available or need to be considered for effective networking?

Adequacy.

Is the I&R service designed to meet the range and magnitude of needs of the intended clientele? Are there ongoing staff training programs for all levels of staff? Are there adequately trained staff and sufficient staff supports to meet service requirements? Do the hardware and software provide ample effectiveness and efficiency to operate a suitable and retrievable automated I&R system?

Accountability.

Is the I&R service responsible to the community, to the agency's board of directors, and to the individual consumer? Do internal procedures assure this accountability? What safeguards for privacy and confidentiality are provided by the I&R agency? Are security measures clearly defined and properly enforced?

Affordability.

Can consumers reach services without undue expense? Can providers finance the basic I&R service with current and projected funding? Can I&R programs continue to operate if or when special project funds are terminated?

Acceptability.

Are people in all socioeconomic groups receptive to I&R as a public service or social utility? Are the inclusive/exclusive criteria clearly defined and strictly adhered to? What exceptions pertain to stated criteria?

Adaptability.

Is the taxonomy indexed to meet the specific level of detail required to identify the specific resource? Is the I&R system sensitive to current social needs and responsive to organizational changes, policy shifts, new legislative mandates, and administrative realignments?

Assessability.

Do well-defined research measures support needed investigation in I&R practice? What measures are taken at what intervals of time to evaluate the I&R agency program? Is the evaluation conducted by outside sources or as a self-study? Are long-term gains as well as short-term benefits taken into account? What are the social costs as well as the fiscal costs in assessing the effectiveness and efficiency of I&R services?

Assured Confidentiality.

What safeguards for privacy and confidentiality are provided by the I&R agency? Are security measures clearly defined and properly enforced? Are there exceptional circumstances in which confidentiality restrictions should be modified?

The above qualities are not weighted according to importance, nor are these items discrete. Rather, it is the combined attributes that represent the essentials of quality practice.

CONCLUSIONS

The vast and diverse field of I&R includes comprehensive services that serve the broad public interest and specialized services that meet individual and family needs. I&R services are also responsive to individual and collective emergency-disaster situations. Given the capability of I&R to provide organized data in accordance with an established taxonomy, and to share databases, an I&R service agency has the capacity to assume a proactive stance in highlighting service needs, advocating change, and introducing innovation. The availability of a national toll-free 211 telephone number will promote universal access to human services at all service levels. Chapter 5 further discusses how I&R can effectively deliver quality services and facilitate improved access to services, as well as how I&R strongly depends upon the structure and managerial aspects of I&R organizations.

REFERENCES

AIRS Directory. (1995–1996). Alliance of Information and Referral Systems, Inc. and United Way of America. *Directory of Information and Referral Services in the United States and Canada.* Joliet, IL: Authors.

Besser, J. (1983). *How to hot line: The Alexandria, Virginia, hot line planning manual.* Alexandria, VA: The Mental Health Association in Alexandria.

Blakely, T. J. (1991). Advocacy in social work. *Information and Referral: The Journal of the Alliance of Information and Referral Systems, 13* (1–2), 19–29.

Bloksberg, L. M., & Caso, E. K. (1967). *Survey of information and referral services existing within the US: Final report.* Waltham, MA: Brandeis University, Florence Heller Graduate School of Advanced Studies in Social Welfare.

Bruni, M. G. (2000). Indexing with the AIRS/INFO LINE Taxonomy of human services. *Information and Referral: The Journal of the Alliance of Information and Referral Systems, 22,* 83–109.

Caplan, G. (1964). *Principles of preventive psychiatry.* New York: Basic Books.

Cueny, D. M. (1999). Correspondence 6/16/99. The Center for Information and Crisis Services. Fl: Lantana. P.O. Box 3588.

Dray, D., Salmers, S., & Larsen, K. (1993). Hurricane Iniki: The ASK-2000 experience. *Information and Referral: The Journal of the Alliance of Information and Referral Systems, 15,* 55–62.

Gandy, N. B. (1993). I&R in times of crisis: The LINC experience. *Information and Referral: The Journal of the Alliance of Information and Referral Systems, 15,* 46–54.

Hogan, M. (1997). Connecticut's experience customizing taxonomy. *AIRS Newsletter, 22*(3), 1.

Interstudy. (1971). *Interviewing and information giving: Working draft.* Minneapolis, MN: Institute for Interdisciplinary Studies of the American Rehabilitation Institute. Information and Referral Centers.

Jacobson, A. (1994). What about confidentiality? When and how to release information. *Information and Referral: The Journal of the Alliance of Information and Referral Systems, 16,* 71–78.

Kahn, A. J., Grossman, L., Bandler, J., Clark, F. R., Galkin, F., & Greenwalt, K. (1966). *Neighborhood information centers: A study and some proposals.* New York: Columbia University School of Social Work.

Kitkowski, L. R. (2000). I&R ethics: Confidentiality and the I&R professional. *AIRS Newsletter, 24* (2), 12.

Laudisio, G. (1993). Disaster aftermath: Redefining response—Hurricane Andrew's impact on I&R. *Information and Referral: The Journal of the Alliance of Information and Referral Systems, 15,* 13–32.

Levinson, R. W., & Liebscher P. (1997). A dynamic I&R partnership: Librarians and social workers. *A National Survey 1997.* AIRS Conference, 1997. Houston, Texas.

Long, N. (1973) Information and Referral Services. A short history and some recommendations. *The Social Service Review, 47* (1), 49–62.

Mass, N. L. (2000). The information and referral interview: Models to remember. *Information and Referral: The Journal of the Alliance of Information and Referral Systems, 22,* 1–62.

Manikowski, D. (2000). Setting inclusion/exclusion criteria: Determining the scope of a resource file. *Information and Referral: The Journal of the Alliance of Information and Referral Systems, 22,* 111–138.

NACAB (2000). National Association of Citizens Advice Bureau. Annual Report. 1998–1999.

Nance, W. (1993). Hurricane Hugo activity report. *Information and Referral: The Journal of the Alliance of Information and Referral Systems, 15,* 1–12.

Roberts, A. R., (Ed.). (1995). *Crisis intervention and time-limited cognitive treatment.* Thousand Oaks, CA: Sage.

Sales, G. (1995). I&R leadership in the information age. *Information and Referral: The Journal of the Alliance of Information and Referral Systems, 17*, 137–150.

Sales, G. (1998). *Disaster services: An excerpt from a taxonomy of human services.* AIRS NERIN Project.

Standards for professional information and referral. (2000). (4th ed.). Seattle, WA: AIRS.

Titmuss, R. M. (1968). *Welfare state and welfare society: In commitment to welfare.* New York: Pantheon Books.

Wallrich, B. (1993). The role of generic I&R in disaster response: INFO LINE of Los Angeles and the civil disturbances of 1992. *Information and Referral: The Journal of the Alliance of Information and Referral Systems, 15,* 33–45.

Wallrich, B. (1998). National disaster project holds promise for AIRS members and their communities. *Information and Referral: The Journal of the Alliance of Information and Referral Systems, 20,* 61–66.

Webster, S. A. (1995). *Disasters and disaster aid. In Encyclopedia of social work* (19th ed., Vol. 1, pp. 761–771). Washington, DC: National Association of Social Workers (NASW) Press.

CHAPTER 5

The Organizational Context of I&R: Diversities and Partnerships

Human service agencies and professionals should not be changed for the sake of using technology. Rather, technology should be adapted to practitioner work patterns, agency and human procedures wherever possible.
Dick Schoech, 1999

T he diversity and complexity of I&R organizational structures defy a neat categorization of I&R agencies. No two I&R organizations are exactly comparable, nor are any two I&R service programs replicable. The size of I&R organizations does not necessarily reflect the size of the population served, nor does the volume of case services indicate the severity of problems that exist in any community. I&R services may range from a one-person, one-phone operation to an extensive statewide or regional computerized program that handles hundreds of calls a day. Even seemingly similar I&R services offered to comparable clientele may vary drastically in range, scope, and quality of services.

Because of these marked variations and the many factors that determine the range and quality of I&R programs, such as funding resources, staffing patterns, and community sanction and support, it is not possible to date to arrive at an ideal or optimal model of I&R operations. Nevertheless, a review of I&R organizations suggests a distinction among agencies that aim to serve universal needs of all people (comprehensive services), organizations that focus on the specific needs of individuals and families (specialized services), and agencies that respond to emergency and disaster conditions. Based on the underpinning concept of I&R as a set of systems, a typology of I&R organizational systems is presented that includes information systems, agency systems, and network systems (see Figure 5.1). However, the initial discussion on I&R organizations will focus on the volume and distribution of I&R agencies within the United States.

I&R AGENCY INVENTORIES

To date, there is neither a comprehensive inventory nor an unduplicated count of the total number of I&R programs, agencies, and networks that exist in the United States. Current reports on the volume of I&R programs tend to represent a gross undercount since a vast number of I&R departments and I&R units that operate within established host agencies are often not identified as I&R services. Thus, many social agencies and public libraries that offer I&R services are not listed in published inventories. Moreover, a growing volume of hot lines, crisis intervention services, self-help groups, and information clearing houses have not been systematically included in existing I&R inventories.

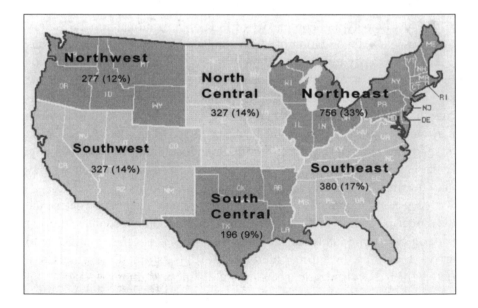

Figure 5.1 Regional distribution of I&R agencies by totals and percentages reported by AIRS in 1995–1996.

Note: Data reported in appendix C.
Source: AIRS Directory 1995–1996.

I&R services are often subsumed under administrative procedures or considered part of an agency intake process. In the absence of a universal, centralized, and reliable inventory it is difficult to identify and to arrive at a reliable estimate on the number of I&R agencies that are currently in operation. However, as the field of I&R continues to regulate its procedures and insists on maintenance of standards and formal accreditation, it is anticipated that far more reliable data on the numbers of I&R agencies will be forthcoming. For purposes of current reporting, however, a membership count from each of the three major national I&R organizations identified collectively as the National I&R TRIAD, is documented in appendices B (1, 2, 3) and C.

REGIONAL DISTRIBUTION OF I&R AGENCIES

As noted on the map of the United States in Figure 5.1, the regional distribution of I&R agencies is reported by totals and percentages and is based on the data reported in the AIRS directory of 1995–1996 (appendices B and C). Appendix B lists the volume of I&R agencies that were reported for each region in 1984–1985 and the comparative data at a later year that apply to each of these three major I&R organizations. Appendix C indicates the comparative I&R data that is reported in the designated regions for the years 1984 and 2000 (as noted, the data reported by each organization reflects a slightly different time period).

As shown on the U.S. map (Figure 5.1), the majority of the I&R agencies are located in the northeast region and make up 33% of all agencies in the nation. The fewest agencies (9%) are located in the south-central region. The southeast indicates 17%, while both the north-central and southwest regions each total 14%, followed by the northwest region at 12%. In a vertical analysis of the regional map, the northeast and southeast regions include exactly half (50%) of all I&R agencies in the nation, whereas the rest of the regions combined comprise the other half of all agencies. Viewing the map horizontally, the northern half of the country includes 60% of the agencies, whereas the southern half includes 40% of all I&R agencies.

The comparative data in appendix C indicate an overall increase in the number of I&R agencies in all regions. However, I&R agencies in the northwest and southeast regions experienced a greater increase. The southwest and south-central regions experienced a marked increase, while the northeast and north-central regions experienced an insignificant increase

TABLE 5.1 Six Highest Ranking States Reported by Total AIRS Agencies and Total Population (1984 & 1995–1996)

State	Region	Total I&R Agencies*		Rank Order of I&R Agencies		Total Population of States** (in millions)	Rank Order of Population
		1984	1995–1996	1984	1995–1996		
California	Southwest	52	181	1	1	27.7	1
Ohio	Northeast	43	124	3	2	10.8	6
Illinois	North Central	31	115	5	3	11.4	5
Texas	South Central	32	111	4.5	4	14.2	3
Pennsylvania	Northeast	32	105	4.5	5	11.9	4
New York	Northeast	45	90	2	6	17.5	2

Sources: *   Directory of Information and Referral Services in the U.S. and Canada. *Alliance of Information and Referral Services, Inc.* (1984–1985). Indianapolis, IN: Author;
Directory of Information and Referral Services. *Alliance of Information and Referral Systems, Inc. and United Way of America* (1995–1996). Joliet, IL: Author.
 **   U.S. Census, 1995 Supplement.

compared to the other regions. In the northeast, for example, the number of I&R agencies in 1984 was 243 and represented 41% of all I&R agencies in the nation. In 1996, however, the total number of agencies in the northeast was 756 and made up only 33% of all agencies in the nation.

A comparison of the six highest ranking states reported by total I&R agencies and total population, indicates that for each of the reporting years (1984 and 1996) there are some shifting of ranks as shown in Table 5.1. California remained number one in rank order in the total number of agencies and total population in1984 and 1996. While New York State has doubled in the number of agencies, the totals of the other five I&R agencies have more than tripled. The changes in rank order indicate that Ohio has moved up from third place in rank order of I&R agencies to second place in 1996. Illinois has also moved up from fifth in rank order to second place. Both Texas and Pennsylvania have remained fourth in rank order. Although New York has doubled in the number of I&R agencies (45–90) in this 12-year period of time, New York ranked sixth in 1995, down from the number two ranking that it held in 1984.

MULTILEVEL I&R AGENCIES

There are enormous variations in the service areas in which I&R services are located and in the nature of clientele whom they serve. It is generally acknowledged that I&R services are dedicated to serve the local community with optimum availability and accessibility. While it may be difficult to define the parameters of a community, it is generally assumed that "community" implies the geographic boundaries of local service areas. I&R services also operate within a variety of jurisdictional units including local counties, townships, cities, states, provinces, and national boundaries. Regional units also vary, depending on whether the I&R agency is operating in an urban, suburban, or rural setting. The I&R program at the Citizens Advice Bureau in Bronx, New York serves a very different population and meets different sets of needs compared to the suburban setting of the I&R program that is conducted at the Middle Country Library in Centereach, Long Island, New York, and certainly unlike the rural community in Arizona described by Alvin Sallee (1985). The remarkable developments in information technology, which have rapidly advanced I&R programs during the decade of the 1990s, have enabled I&R services to function at all levels of operation and with various combinations of city, state, regional, provincial, national, and international I&R programs.

AUSPICES

The auspices of I&R agencies vary depending on whether they are public agencies, private agencies, voluntary nonprofit or for-profit organizations. The application of I&R standards as formulated in the current Standards (2000) and the federal approval of the 211 universal telephone service have called attention to the vital role of the federal government in I&R policy (Sales, 1995). The advent of military-based I&R programs since the early 1980s has also significantly increased the role of the federal government in I&R operations. State and regional I&R associations have dramatically expanded I&R activities within the parameters of their respective organizations. Though it is difficult to ascertain the volume of I&R services in the private sector, there is increased recognition of the expanding role of the for-profit sector in the growth of I&R programs. The Private Practice Referral Services of the Massachusetts chapter of the National Association of Social Workers used the I&R service to "engage prospective clients" (AIRS 1993). The Red Book, Directory of Services for the Lower Mainland (1998) in Canada includes both public and private agency listings. As noted in this directory, "the principal criterion for including an agency is that it is either an ongoing nonprofit operation providing a direct service to the public, or a proprietary agency providing a unique service." This directory also provides a special section on "Private Practitioners Pages," which lists licensed counselors, therapists, and psychologists who pay a fee to the I&R agency for inclusion in the directory.

I&R services are also available in a wide variety of agency settings on all levels of operation as reported in volume 19 of the AIRS journal (1997) in the special edition entitled "The Many Faces of I&R." I&R agencies may operate independently in local kiosks or in community institutions, such as libraries, hospitals, schools, and churches. State and federal I&R programs may represent independent I&R programs or I&R networks. Since I&R agencies represent mixed types and unique hybrids of organizational structures, it is difficult to delineate discrete types of I&R organizations. In an effort to arrive at a categorization of widely diversified organizational structures, a typology of I&R systems is presented which suggests five models of I&R organizations.

A TYPOLOGY OF I&R SYSTEMS

The following typology of five I&R systems (Figure 5.2) is designed to delineate significant differences among various types of I&R agency sys-

tems in diversified settings. The first category represents informational
I&R service systems, such as the clearinghouse that reports on a vast array
of health disorders, (e.g., cancer, alcohol, substance abuse, and kidney
disorders). Other informational services report on hot lines, self-help
groups, and emergency services. The second category designates an independent or freestanding I&R agency system as represented by public
kiosks. A third type of an I&R agency is located within a host agency and
therefore functions as an interagency and intra-agency system such as the
public library or a social service agency. A decentralized network constitutes a fourth type of agency system that operates its own I&R system
within a designated area in which other agencies may or may not provide
I&R services. A fifth type of organization is a centralized I&R network
that is conducted within a fully coordinated I&R system, and includes
member agency units that relate to one central I&R facility, such as the
Connecticut State I&R program. An overview of the selected organizations represented by the configurations of each of the corresponding I&R
systems is shown in Figure 5.2.

I&R INFORMATION SYSTEMS

I&R service systems that operate primarily as information and crisis intervention systems transmit and impart information from various databases
through a variety of media, including telephone services, hot lines, clearinghouses, published directories, radio, and television (both network and
cable). During the 1970s there was a dramatic expansion of prerecorded
telephone informational services relating to health and legal services. The
fastest growing of these phone-based services has been Tel-Med's telephone cassette libraries on health information, which enables an anony-
mous caller to receive medically approved information by listening to taped
messages on prerecorded cassettes.

Tel-Med began in 1972 as an experiment in community medical information under the auspices of the San Bernardino County Medical Society.
Within 5 years, more than 100 cities had a Tel-Med program, and by 1990
there were more than 250 programs operating in 43 states and averaging
more than a million calls per month. The original tape library of 50 topics has increased to 335 tapes in the master library, many of which have
been translated into Spanish. Tel-Med systems have also been incorporated in existing I&R programs. For example, the statewide information
and referral system of the North Carolina Department of Human Resources,

TYPES OF I&R SYSTEMS	DESCRIPTION OF TYPES OF I&R SYSTEMS	CONFIGURATION	TYPE OF ORGANIZATION
I INFORMATIONAL I&R SYSTEMS	*An Informational I&R System* provides information-assistance to all inquirers (phone, walk-in, e-mail, Internet, or correspondence).	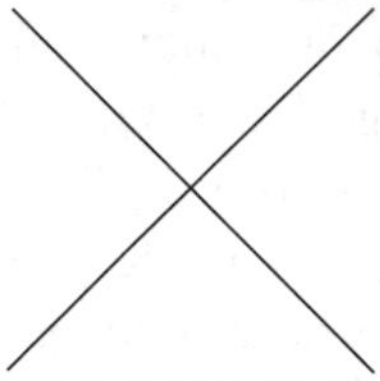	Clearing Houses
II FREESTANDING I&R SYSTEMS	*A Freestanding I&R Agency System* operates independently and autonomously. I&R is the single, generic service provided to the public.	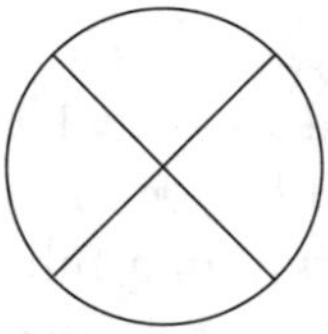	Kiosks
III INTRA-AGENCY I&R SYSTEMS	An *Intra-agency I&R Subsystem* operates as an I&R department or unit within the host agency in which it is based.	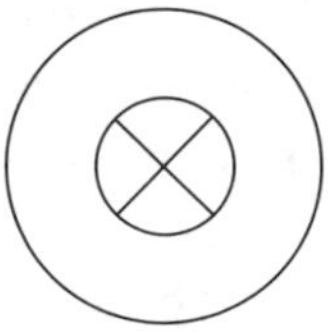	Public Libraries
IV DECENTRALIZED I&R NETWORKS	A *Decentralized I&R Network* includes multiple I&R agencies in designated service areas that may or may not link up with other I&R agencies.	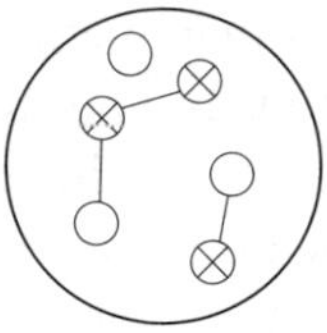	Military Installations
V CENTRALIZED I&R NETWORKS	A *Centralized I&R Network* includes multiple I&R agencies in a designated service area that are directly accountable to a single generic I&R agency or to a regional alliance.	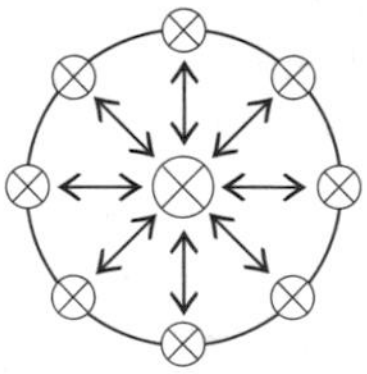	I&R State Systems Regional Alliances

Figure 5.2 A typology of I&R organizational systems.

LEGEND:

   ✕ I&R Information System;

   ◯ Social Agency;

   ⊗ I&R Agency System.

known as Call-Line, provides Tel-Med services as part of its I&R program on social services, as does Info-Line in Akron, Ohio. In Rhode Island, the Information Services of the Council for Community Services incorporated Tel-Med into its I&R system and has provided social work services on a 24-hour-a-day basis as a follow-up to Tel-Med referrals.

Another taped telephone message system, referred to as Tel-Law, has also been developed for legal information. Tape-recorded messages provide general information on the legal system and more specialized information on such topics as estate planning, adoption, bankruptcy, consumer affairs, separation, and divorce. A lawyer referral information service refers inquirers with legal problems to qualified lawyers through telephone-taped messages according to convenient geographic locations or by specific area of legal specialization.

To cover crisis calls that are received after regular office hours, a growing number of social agencies arrange to transfer callers to other I&R services that operate beyond the usual office hours. A popular type of crisis service is the hot line, a telephone service that may be staffed by volunteers who are trained to respond to emergencies. Hot-line staff may also be composed of peer-group members, who are considered to have special understanding and empathy with the callers. The growing numbers of hot lines indicate the pressing needs of people in crises or perceived crisis situations to obtain information and reach helping services without undue delay. A hot-line request may entail a single contact or more extensive contacts between the client and the I&R agent. In either case, hot lines usually rely on effective working relationships with human service organizations that can respond under emergency conditions and can provide time-limited treatment. A National Directory of Crisis Hotlines lists categories of hot lines that include toll-free crisis hot lines, hot lines that relate to addiction, victim services, witness-assistance programs, and battered women and children (Roberts, 1995).

Clearinghouses have become important information sources since the 1960s, when federal human service programs proliferated rapidly and often with nontraditional service delivery patterns. Clearinghouses may provide telephone informational services as well as published directories that inventory extensive volumes of human services, often of special interest to the homebound and to persons living alone. To assist the consumer with inquiries that pertain to information on federal government resources, Federal Information Centers (FICs) have been established to respond primarily to questions about resources that operate on a federal level. The FIC program was established by a directive of President Lyndon Johnson in 1965 and has expanded to respond to a wide range of inquiries that may pertain to veterans benefits, social security, immigration and naturalization, patents, copyrights, tax assistance, wage and hour laws, job information, and Medicare. Every state in the United States has at least one or more FICs and many FICs work cooperatively with existing I&R agencies.

FREESTANDING I&R SYSTEMS: KIOSKS

A freestanding I&R agency is the public kiosk which provides information for the general public regarding areas of special interest to inquirers. The AIRS standards define a kiosk as "a freestanding structure, often located in malls or other public places, which houses community resource information that people can access without outside assistance." Interest in kiosks has mounted as technology has provided increased opportunity for the public-at-large to obtain information at "kiosks," which are locally accessible and lodged in a convenient boxlike computerized structure for public use. The kiosk is especially designed for people who can easily access information that pertains to local community resources. Another function of the kiosk system is the Community Resource Directory System, which concurrently collects demographic information and service profiles from kiosk users with an aim to acquire information on service requests in order to help community planners to understand the community and its needs.

The county of DuPage in Wheaton, Illinois, introduced the Community Resource Information System and advertised in its local newspaper (Edware, 1999) that the "grocery list of the future will include milk, eggs, and counseling services via its kiosk." In addition to listing "thousands" of human service agencies, kiosks also provide information on local job openings, volunteer opportunities, child care options, and information about local businesses. It is expected that the popularity of kiosks will increase given the simplicity of the touch system with which it can be operated by the consumer (Lawrence, 1999). Another example of an operating kiosk is the Resource House, which can be accessed on the Internet (www.iowaresourcenetwork.com), to reach a wide variety of information sources that include public schools, community health alliances, housing choices, and the disaster program of the American Red Cross (United Way of Lake County, 2000).

INTRA-AGENCY I&R SYSTEMS: PUBLIC LIBRARIES

I&R agencies that operate within host agencies represent highly diversified structural and functional patterns of I&R programs. These I&R agencies include agency intake departments, emergency services, crisis intervention centers, and mobile services. These I&R services also frequently operate as an auxiliary service within a host social service organization, such as public welfare agencies, mental health centers, family and child welfare agencies, and other human service organizations. Hospitals and schools also indicate increased involvement with I&R programs within their community institutions, and may function as a supplementary or complementary service to promote the primary goals of health care and education.

With the advent of the 1970s, I&R programs began to proliferate in public libraries. The rationale for this proliferation appears logical, particularly in view of the many attractive features that the public library provides for I&R program development. The public library is traditionally revered as the storehouse of all recorded information. As a well-recognized and highly respected community institution, the public library offers a uniquely suitable setting for needed information, referral, and a wide range of helping services. The public library also provides a highly convenient and accessible location for universal access to I&R services. Moreover, the local library offers a cost-free public service and is traditionally regarded as a nonpolitical facility. As for availability, the library is usually open for services at various times during evenings and weekends that exceed the more limited hours of most social services agencies. Libraries also offer an array of special helping services by providing talking books, large print books, and assistive devices for people who are visually limited and hearing impaired. Not to be overlooked is the important role of librarians as trained information specialists. Recognizing this importance, the community section of the Public Library Association (PLA, 1997) developed its own guidelines for I&R services in the public library.

Reports on I&R services in public libraries did not appear until the early 1970s when the Detroit Public Library established an I&R service known as TIP (The Information Place). An early formulation of the TIP service was presented by Jones (1978). TIP has continued to be a leader in the I&R field in view of its community involvement in database networks and research reports in telephone technology and the taxonomy. Other library-based I&R programs have been identified with their particular acronyms including the Neighborhood Information Center (NIC) in Houston, and the Library Information Center in Memphis. Individual libraries and total library systems have implemented highly differentiated I&R programs.

From 1970 to the mid-1980s, library-based I&R programs continued to expand. Childers' survey of Information and Referral Services (1984) presented models of I&R-based programs in selected libraries. Childers concluded that public libraries will continue to expand with highly differentiated models of I&R programs. Childers' determining criteria of the seven libraries under study were a representation of differences in locale or setting, the nature of clientele, the use of manual- or computer-based operations, and the role of I&R both as a direct service and as a support service to other agencies.

In addition to the operation of the library-based I&R programs, public libraries have also become centers of organizational networks and share common databases with member agencies. With funding and encouragement from the Skillman Foundation (AIRS, 1999), TIP in Detroit, Michigan, manages the central resource database used by major I&R providers. The library's database serves Wayne County as well as other out-of-county resource organizations such as United Way, Tel-Help, and the Child Care Coordinating Council.

Another case in point in library databases is the Community Resource Database of Long Island, located at the Middle Country Library, Centereach, Long Island. The Community Resource Database of Long Island offers individuals and families easy access to resource information with special interest in promoting the health and welfare of children and families (CRD, 1999). Although public libraries provide direct I&R services within local communities, public libraries are also involved in building shared databases beyond the service boundaries of the local community. This interdisciplinary model of professional collaboration suggests new opportunities for shared service delivery and the use of centralized databases for community planning and programming (Levinson, 1996).

A national survey was conducted in 1996–1997 by Levinson and Liebscher to ascertain the extent to which public libraries and social agencies are aware of one another's service programs within a given community and to assess the degree to which these service organizations cooperate in the provision of I&R services at the local level. A study sample of 200 libraries and 211 social agencies located within the same geographic area were selected. The goal of the study was to ascertain the extent to which public libraries and social services are aware of one another's existence within a given locale. A second goal was to assess the degree to which these two kinds of organizations cooperate in the provision of I&R services at the local level. The third goal of the survey was to raise the level of mutual awareness and to promote linkages between public libraries and social agencies in the provision of I&R services. Survey findings indicated that while more social agencies utilize public library services with increased frequency, librarians have also broadened their service agendas to include I&R services that are focused on the enhancement of family life and the promotion of health and mental health for all age groups. An interdisciplinary model involving social workers and librarians in public libraries and known as Senior Connections, is discussed extensively in chapter 8.

DECENTRALIZED I&R NETWORKS: THE MILITARY

A decentralized I&R system generally denotes an I&R program that operates independently but which may or may not be connected with other I&R agencies within the local community. Military installations are unique in that these military bases are members of an international system of military-based services, while simultaneously aware of I&R resources that may operate within the broader community in which the military base is located. Thus, the military community can operate its own home-based I&R system while also relating to the I&R programs within the community in which the military personnel and family members reside.

The military Family Support Centers (FSCs), which were initiated in the mid-1960s, focused on the needs of the military to maintain positive family relationships whether living with their families on base or deployed in active service. The centers called attention to problems of child abuse, domestic violence, employment of spouses, and teenage family conflicts. They are staffed by army personnel, civilians, and volunteers who are committed to provide support and assistance to the military and to their families. Relocation of military personnel, which occurs every 2 to 3 years, requires a constant need to learn about new resources and services in each new community (Goldstein, 1985). The FSCs totaled 297 in 1996 and existed in the army, the navy, the air force, the marine core, and the coast guard. Some of the core functions and services provided at most centers are I&R, financial, mental health, family life education, wellness, and readiness programs.

A telecommunications system known as FAMNET links every air force FSC to base line programs. The goal is to provide proactive prevention-based programs, which are targeted to alleviate and minimize family stress caused by the demands of military life. Robert Fuller, chief executive officer of human resources development, has introduced FAMNET Crossroads as the information system to a world of military topics ranging from employment, to financial assistance, and to services for teens. For purposes of providing information to the military, the following databases are available:

(a)   Military Children & Youth,
(b)   Military Family Resource Center,
(c)   Military Teens on the Move, and
(d)   Standard Installation Topic Exchange Service.

During the 2000 AIRS conference, it was announced that all branches of the armed services are currently represented in the AIRS membership. As corporate members of AIRS, military and civilian personnel at military bases seek to professionalize themselves by qualifying for the position of the certified I&R specialist. Military versions of AIRS standards have been adapted to meet the special qualification for I&R specialists in the armed services. Since the mid-1980s, military personnel have assumed an increasingly vital role in participating in workshops and training sessions at the annual AIRS conferences (Strickland, 2000).

The U.S. military personnel of the 1990s is markedly different from earlier years. Military couples tend to marry earlier, become parents at a younger age, and have more children (Black, 1993). Unlike former family patterns, military personnel make efforts to balance careers and child care in the face of relocations and separations. Military families currently outnumber single service members with a ratio of 60% married compared with 40% single.

The most dramatic change in military families during the 1980s and 1990s has been the increase in the numbers of employed military spouses. The entry of women into the military has created a new breed of a military marriage, which is referred to as *the joint service marriage*. Aware of the needs of these varying family constellations, Anne Tarzier, Office of Deputy Assistant Secretary of Defense, Military Community and Family

Policy, has specified three major goals for military families: (a) positive family functioning, (b) economic management, and (c) the well-being of children and youth. Given these new and complex family strains in the face of the military priorities of "deployment and family readiness," availability of I&R services has proved to be of special importance to families of military personnel.

CENTRALIZED I&R NETWORKS: STATE SYSTEMS AND REGIONAL ALLIANCES

A centralized network is usually created when a single agency assumes the responsibility of sharing I&R services with member agencies within a defined state or region. State and regional associations of I&R agencies represent organizational networks that share programs, databases, training sessions, and joint planning. The Connecticut I&R system is in effect a state program, totally involved with state government, and has distinguished itself as a centralized network. With facilitation from the state government, Connecticut has also effectively achieved the establishment of the 211 universal telephone service. Another level of networking is the regional level, which may involve a single state or may include regions that border several states. The regional associations are usually identified with the names of the individual state or states in which they reside.

As listed in the AIRS 1995–1996 directory, there are 19 regional associations that represent I&R organizations within individual states such as FLAIRS in Florida, CAIRS in California, PAIRS in Pennsylvania, TAIRS in Texas, and NYSAIRS in New York. These 19 agencies arrange annual and semiannual meetings to discuss topics of interest to the member agencies. Training sessions are planned with a view toward advancing the expertise of the agency personnel. Common areas of interest vary according to the specific priorities that are pertinent at any given time, (e.g., advances in technology, updating of databases, indexing of the taxonomy, and instituting the 211 universal telephone service). The regional alliances provide opportunity for greater impact of I&R systems on behalf of individual agencies as well as for state-wide dissemination. The regional associations set aside special meetings at the annual AIRS conferences to review their agendas, to consult with members of other associations, and to reinforce the momentum that derives from common interests in circumscribed geographic areas.

NETWORKING STRATEGIES

A network denotes a constellation of multiple I&R systems that operate information and referral programs within a defined service area or share a mutual area of interest. Because the benefits of networking have gained increased recognition as cost-efficient as well as service-effective, a variety of linkages have developed within I&R agencies. The following strategies promote I&R networking as outlined in Table 5.2.

ORGANIZATIONAL STRATEGIES

The national I&R TRIAD represents I&R networking of three major organizations in the interest of promoting I&R programs that have been initiated and subsequently adopted by each of the three organizations, as discussed in Chapter 2. The location and colocation of I&R programs in

TABLE 5.2 Strategies for I&R Networking

Organizational Strategies
- Interorganizational mandates, contracts, and agreements
- Location and colocation of I&R programs
- Staffing and training
- Multiple funding/joint financing
- Outreach and public relations

Service Strategies
- The AIRS/INFO LINE Taxonomy—A common language
- Centralized resource inventories
- Linkages of generic and specialized I&R services
- Collaborative and complementary services
- Adherence to I&R standards

Policy and Planning Strategies
- Political support
- Joint research and evaluation
- Interagency planning

Technology Strategies
- Database sharing
- Listservs, e-mail, telecommunications (211)
- Dissemination via the Internet

Adaptation of Source: Levinson, R. W. (1988). *Information and Referral Networks: Doorways to Human Services.* New York: Springer Publishing.

community institutions, such as schools, libraries, and churches, provide a strategy for organizational networking. Staffing and training programs are often provided by special staff on a consultation basis across several I&R organizations. One of the most effective strategies that promotes networking is the granting of multiple funding or joint financing of selective I&R programs. Joint I&R programs in public relations can be more effective in incurring less costs and gaining more visibility when presented by a network of I&R organizations.

SERVICE STRATEGIES

The AIRS/INFO LINE Taxonomy, which was initiated by LA Info/Line and subsequently adopted by AIRS and United Way of America (UWA), has been accepted as a universal classification system. The taxonomy serves as an effective networking instrument for all operating I&R agencies.

In the process of database sharing, I&R agencies can develop cooperative working relationships and thereby avoid duplication of effort and gaps in services. Linkages of generic and specialized I&R services can provide networks to facilitate maximum utilization of existing resources. Collaborative and complementary services can facilitate the ability of people who need services to find the most appropriate provider. The professionalization of I&R standards as formulated in the fourth edition (2000) of the AIRS standards suggests effective networking on all levels of operations including local, state or provincial, regional, national, and international levels.

POLICY AND PLANNING STRATEGIES

One of the most salient lesson that has been learned from the experience of promoting the 211 universal telephone service is that a primary reason for success in the 211 approval process has been the effective networking of the participating agencies in the 211 system. Joint research, evaluation, and planning are most successful in the operation of I&R agency networks that share common areas of interest.

A report of crisis networks known as NERIN and INFORM are made up of highly diversified agencies (Aberg, 1997). NERIN is a partnership with multiple organizations such as Federal Emergency Management Agency, UWA, Life Line, and American Red Cross (ARC). Similarly, a list of INFORM members includes a mix of voluntary and public agencies such as the American Society of Suicidology, National Association of Child Care Resource and Referral Agencies, and the American Library Association. AIRS memberships in these organizational networks have created new opportunities to extend disaster services and meet emergencies in a timely manner.

The effectiveness of networking is critically dependent upon the quality of leadership and the competency of staff in establishing organizational linkages as well as the availability of appropriate technology. Networking is often a deliberate, sensitive political process of achieving effective working relationships among diverse agencies, each of which is involved in its own interests and organizational maintenance. According to Haynes and Mickelson (1997), the process of networking and coalition building requires that "all aspects of a given issue be carefully examined to identify points of potential commonality." The coalition process that led to the approval of the 211 universal telephone service is a case-in-point. The strategies involved a clarification of the problem, a declaration of need, and a proposed plan that documented the desired benefits to be gained. The benefactors included the agencies, the legislators, and most directly, the clientele. Thus, the 211 success was essentially a coalition building process.

TECHNOLOGY STRATEGIES

With the technological advancements in computers and information handling, significant gains can be accomplished in organizing efforts toward networking. Coalition building can be effectively expedited using fax machines, e-mail communication, cellular telephones, listservs, and the Internet (Schoech, 1999). In addition to data communication with experts around the world, members of a coalition can communicate in a matter of seconds for a fraction of the costs of mailings. Keeping people informed and connected can be critical factors in organizing others and influencing policymakers.

The parameters of I&R networks may be determined by geographic proximity, by funding sources, or by jurisdictional boundaries. However, I&R services that are restricted to the specific jurisdictional boundaries of cities, towns, or villages do not necessarily receive funding from these governing bodies, but nevertheless share commonalities. I&R networks have also developed within national organizations such as the Easter Seal Society and the American Red Cross, which maintain local chapters that carry out the organization's I&R programs at the local level. Some of the multifunction service centers that evolved as a locality-specific I&R service network during the 1960s aimed to help clients connect with an array of available services. However, some of the services within the center functioned as discrete units, usually as outposts or satellites of larger organizations. Nevertheless, the multiservice center represents a potentially effective model of a one-stop center that is capable of offering a cafeteria of services to the inquiring client and of providing a coordinated and well-integrated I&R network.

ACCREDITATION

The quality of I&R services can be difficult to challenge in the absence of a national regulatory and accrediting body. In the past, individual I&R agencies have developed their own self-evaluation instruments to test agency performance. Since the early 1970s, accreditation has been a major concern of I&R agencies in establishing I&R as a professional service. However, it was not until 1997 that AIRS published an Accreditation Application which requires a two-phase operation: (a) consultation, and (b) on-site reviews. AIRS outlined the phasing of the accreditation process, which is available to all requesting member agencies, regardless of size or scope of service. The accreditation procedure is formatted to state the accreditation standard and then to inquire whether the agency meets the specific standard. During the initial *consultation phase* the agency confers with one of the review team members, who acts as a liaison to the agency under review. Following this phase, an on-site review is conducted to ascertain whether the agency is satisfactorily meeting the accreditation standards in the following areas: Organizational Structure, Personnel Administration, Training/Orientation, Service Delivery, and Program Evaluation. When AIRS published its *Accreditation Application*, a specific requirement held that "annual measurable program goals and objectives" are to be included for the current year plus a comparison to the evaluation of prior years (AIRS Accreditation Application, 1997).

Although an accreditation application was not formally available from AIRS until 1997, the urgency of instituting the accreditation process was fully recognized by Ann Jacobson, the chairperson of the AIRS standards and accreditation committee in 1985. According to Jacobson (1985), the system of accreditation signifies that the agency is exercising a high degree of "social responsibility and self-imposed quality controls." To the community, accreditation signifies that a service is being rendered with competence and that funds are being employed for valid social purposes. Since accreditation is a continuous process, not a one-time phenomenon, it signifies the agency's intention to aim toward "ever higher goals of effectiveness."

COSTS AND FINANCING

What constitutes adequate funding depends upon the range, scope, staffing, and parameters of the I&R service. It is difficult to ascertain the costs of I&R services in the absence of standardized units of services and centralized data reporting systems. A financial study by Hohenstein and Banks (1975) estimated that the cost per service ranged from $3.50 in a metropolitan area, using a large number of volunteers, to approximately $34.00 in a small community with all paid staff. The observed median cost per service request was established at $7.86. In identifying the cost of I&R on a per-unit service basis, differential utilization of volunteer staff time was considered to be the critical factor. At this early stage of I&R program development the following questions were asked: Are volunteers used as receptionists, resource specialists, or counselors? If trained volunteers are engaged in direct client contact, are the costs of supervision and training programs taken into consideration? In arriving at I&R costs, are the volume and type of requests handled taken into account? Are walk-in services more costly than telephone services, since more staff time is required to serve clients by personal contact?

On the issue of cost benefit analysis of case outcomes, another financial study, sponsored by the Administration on Aging (AoA) and conducted by Cooper and Company (1985), concluded that there was no clear evidence of significant differences in productivity or labor costs between walk-in services and telephone services. Another finding of this study was that age-integrated services may be less costly to operate than age-segregated agencies. Since 1985 there has been a dearth of published financial studies of I&R organizations. The lack of a common language has been a limitation in the uniform definitions of services. Furthermore, the diversity of I&R operations within the existing agencies are reported with enormous variations, and therefore preclude comparable agency studies within a similar time period.

The majority of I&R systems are dependent upon multiple funding sources from public, voluntary, and proprietary sectors. Federal, state, and local funding allocations tend to vary enormously from one fiscal year to another. As noted in Table 5.3, the public sources for the funding for I&R programs constitute almost 45% of all I&R funding that is derived from federal, state, and local government sources. Federal funding constitutes almost 17% of public funding with allocations for the I&R programs for the military and AoA. Funding from private nonprofit sources represents 28%, which includes donations, good and services, foundations, and sectarian sources. In the voluntary sector, UWA emerges as the major supporter of voluntary funds (27.21%), thereby representing over a quarter of all funding allocated to I&R programs (Key, 2000).

As I&R programs have expanded into major financial enterprises, since the decade of the 1990s there has been a marked expansion in the size of budgets. Above is a listing of budgetary data that were included in the annual reports of these six selected agencies within the years from 1997 to 1999. The budgets in Table 5.4 range from nearly half a million to a grand sum of more than $65 million. Three of the agency budgets range between one and a quarter million to one and three quarters of a million dollars. One agency has a budget of more than $4 million. The mounting

TABLE 5.3 Funding Sources for I&R Programs

TYPE AGENCY	TOTALS	Percentages
Voluntary	**357**	**27.21%**
United Way	357	27.21%
Public	**590**	**44.97%**
Federal Government	220	16.77%
State Government	189	14.41%
Local Government	181	13.80%
Private Nonprofit	**365**	**27.82%**
Donations	146	11.13%
Goods & Services	134	10.21%
Foundations	78	5.95%
Sectarian Agencies	7	0.53%
GRAND TOTAL	**1,312**	**100.00%**

Source: Directory of Information & Referral Services in the United States and Canada. *Alliance of Information & Referral Systems, Inc. & United Way of America* (1995–1996).

TABLE 5.4 Budgetary Data Reported by Six I&R Agencies

Name of Agency	Location	Web Site	Budget Year	Budget in $
1 Philadelphia Corporation for Aging (PCA)	Philadelphia, PA	www.pcaphl.org	1998	65,075,790
2 Texas Council for Developmental Disabilities	Austin, TX	www.rehab.state.tx.us	1999	4,220,588
3 Community Information Toronto (CIT)	Toronto, Canada	www.communityinfotoronto.org	1998	1,832,237
4 United Way of Metropolitan Atlanta	Atlanta, GA	www.unitedwayatl.org	1997–1998	1,389,695
5 Information & Referral Services	Tucson, AZ	www.azstarnet.com/azinfo	1998	1,270,008
6 FIRST—Family Information & Referral Service Teams, Inc.	White Plains, NY	www.firstwp.org	1997	427,949

Source: Data based on annual reports submitted by agencies in mail survey (1998–1999).

sums of current budget reports, which appear significantly higher than earlier years, suggest that I&R has become a major "information industry" with involvement in the public, voluntary nonprofit, and for-profit sectors.

Some assurance of adequate funding for start-up and maintenance of I&R services is critical to organizational survival. Many an attempt to initiate an I&R program has failed because of lack of adequate funds to meet the costs required to operate a projected I&R service. The majority of I&R systems are dependent upon multiple funding sources from the public, voluntary, and proprietary sectors. In view of the high level of technological development, the costs of I&R operations have increased dramatically within the past 10 years. Since the purchasing of hardware and software is a major expense in every I&R program, a comprehensive knowledge of the technology and the costs involved are critical.

CONCLUSIONS

Over the past 40 years, dating back to the social programs of the 1960s and the Older Americans Act of 1965, there has been a continuous expansion of I&R services that became far more extensive in the decade of the 1990s. While I&R programs have been able to chart new networks and formulate new partnerships in diverse organizational settings, the focus on access to services in the local community has remained paramount, including the local public library, kiosks, and the community-based telephone service available at the 211 telephone number. In view of the special challenges for I&R provision, given the current and projected expansion of the aging population, the following chapter 6 is an analysis and a justification for a "seamless I&R service system" for older adults as well as for persons of all ages.

REFERENCES

Aberg, P. (1997, April/May). From the executive director. *AIRS Newsletter, 22* (1), 10–11.

AIRS. (1993). Making the connection: Engaging prospective clients in the referral process. *Information and Referral: The Journal of the Alliance of Information and Referral Systems, 15,* 114–126.

AIRS. (1997). Special edition: The many faces of I&R. *Information & Referral: The Journal of the Alliance of Information and Referral Systems, 19.*

AIRS. (1999, August/September). Detroit's Skillman Foundation presented with AIRS 1999 Distinguished Service Award. *AIRS Newsletter, 24* (1), 1.

AIRS Accreditation Application. (1997). *Alliance of Information and Referral Systems, Inc.* Seattle, WA: Author.

Black, W. G., Jr. (1993). Military-induced family separation: A stress reduction intervention. *Social Work, 38* (3), 273–280.

Childers, T. (1984). *Information and referral: Public libraries.* Norwood, NJ: Ablex Publishing Corporation.

Cooper and Company. (1985). *Costs and benefits of information and referral under "The Older Americans Act."* Administration on Aging, Office of Human Development, Department of Health, Education and Welfare. Washington, DC: Department of Health, Education, and Welfare.

CRD. (1999). Community Resource Database of Long Island Expansion Phase Year 2 (1998–1999): *Final Progress Report to the Long Island Community Foundation.* August 1999. Middle Country Library Foundation.

Edware, C. H. (1999, February 9). Need social services? Go to the store. *The Daily Herald.*

Goldstein, F. L. (1985). Development and evaluation of a worldwide information and referral system: The history of air force family programs. *Information and Referral: The Journal of the Alliance of Information and Referral Systems, 7* (2), 34–50.

Haynes, K. S., & Mickelson, J. (1997). *Affecting change: Social workers in the political arena* (3rd ed.). White Plains, NY: Longman.

Hohenstein, C. L., & Banks, J. (1975). *I&R program configuration: A guide for a statewide planning* (DHEW Pub. No. (OHD) 76-20114). Washington, DC: United States Department of Health, Education, and Welfare.

Jacobson, A. (1985). Why accreditation? *AIRS Newsletter, 13* (9), 7–8.

Jones, C. S. (Ed.). (1978). *Public library information and referral services.* Syracuse, NY: Gaylord.

Key, K. H. (2000). *Democratizing access to human services information: Positioning United Way.* Alexandria, VA: United Way of America.

Lawrence, J. (1999, September 14). September 14th, Information may be as near as your grocer. *Chicago Tribune.* Metro Lake.

Levinson, R. W. (1996). Expanding I&R services for older adults in public libraries: Senior Connections (1984–1995). *Information and Referral: The Journal of the Alliance of Information and Referral Systems, 18,* 21–40.

PLA. (1997). American Library Association. Public Library Association. Community Information Section. *Guidelines for establishing community information and referral services in public libraries: With a selectively annotated guide to the literature of community information & referral* (4th ed.). Chicago, IL: ALA. PLA.

The Red Book, Directory of Services for the Lower Mainland. (1998). *Special section: Private practitioner's pages* (pp. 931–1021). Information Services, Vancouver.

Roberts, A. R. (Ed.). (1995). *Crisis intervention and time-limited cognitive treatment*. National Directory of Crisis Hot Lines (pp. 333–419). Thousand Oaks, CA: SAGE.

Sales, G. (1995). The role of information and referral in the national information infrastructure: An AIRS position paper. In *Out of the shadows: Information & referral, bringing people and services together* (pp. 12–16). Joliet, IL: AIRS.

Sallee, A. (1985). An agricultural extension model for information and referral rural outreach. *Information & Referral: The Journal of the Alliance of Information and Referral Systems, 7* (2), 17–33.

Schoech, D. (1999). *Human services technology*. Binghamton, NY: The Haworth Press.

Standards for professional information and referral (2000). (4th ed.). Seattle, WA: AIRS.

Strickland, G. (2000, April). Military I&R—A horse of a different color. *AIRS Newsletter*, p. 5.

United Way of Lake County. (2000, Winter). Kiosks prove to be a big hit. *Community Connections*, p. 3.

CHAPTER 6

New I&R Challenges in an Expanding Aging Society

We are in a real transition from what I have called the
modern aging of the 1930s to the 1990s, to a new aging
that will reveal itself over the next 10 to 20 years and
will mean a whole new approach to aging and being old.
Fernando M. Torres-Gil, 2001

WHY A SPECIAL CHAPTER ON AGING AND I&R?

The aging constitute the fastest growing population group in society today and will continue to expand in the 21st century with a host of diverse needs and new demands for I&R services. In viewing the field of I&R since its origin in the mid-1960s, the involvement of the national Administration on Aging (AoA) in I&R research and program development has been a driving force in the expansion of I&R services in the United States. As specified in the Older Americans Act (OAA) of 1965, I&R is a universally mandated service for all older Americans on federal, state and local levels and operates under the auspices of the AoA. It is also noteworthy that a national computerized I&R telephone system, known as the Eldercare Locator, which is in operation under the auspices of the National Association State Units on Aging (NASUA), responds to requests for I&R services that are targeted to serve the aging and their caregivers. Because of the dramatic expansion of older persons in the United States and throughout the world, attention to the needs of older persons is imperative, including the need for convenient access to information and referral services.

DEMOGRAPHICS AND DIVERSITY

Older Americans are increasing both in numbers and in proportion to the total population. The older population consisting of persons 65 and over numbered 34.1 million in 1997, which represented 12.7% of the U.S. population or about one in every eight Americans. As noted in Figure 6.1, the percentage of Americans 65+ has more than tripled (4.1% in 1900 to 12.7% in 1997), and the total number has increased from 3.1 million to 34.1 million. The average life expectancy has also increased significantly, with an additional 17.6 years, 19.0 years for females and 15.8 years for males (Profiles, 1998).

Looking ahead, the older population will continue to grow significantly in the future. As seen in Figure 6.1, the population will burgeon between the years 2010 and 2030 when the baby-boom generation reaches age 65. In fact, it has been projected that by 2030, the older population will number 70 million older persons, which represents more than twice their number in 1997. This phenomenal increase of older persons is referred to by Dychtwald and Flower (1989) as "an evolving gerontocracy." Chronologically,

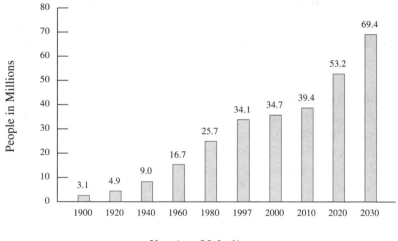

Year (as of July 1)

Figure 6.1 Number of persons 65+ (1900 to 2030).

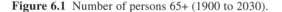

Note: Increments in years on horizontal scale are uneven. *Based on data from U.S. Bureau of the Census*
Source: "A Profile of Older Americans." (1998). *American Association of Retired Persons,* p. 2.

the older population itself is aging. Based on census data reported in 1996, a dramatic increase is expected among centenarians, as 1 in 26 of the baby boomers is due to reach more than 100 years (Hooyman & Kiyak, 1996). In projecting future population growth, minority populations are expected to represent 25% of the population of older people in 2030, up from 15% in 1997. These trends indicate that the population of older people will become more diversified as a greater proportion will be non-White. According to Torres-Gil (1992), the U.S. population will be a nation of older, more diverse, complex groups with a declining population of youths. As indicated in Figure 6.2, it is projected that during the successive decades of 1990 to 2020, ethnic minority older persons (age 65+) will increase significantly among the following groups: Asian and Pacific Islanders (358%); the Hispanic (300%); the American Indian, Eskimo and Aleut Groups (150%); and the Black population (102%). The least increase (58%) is projected for White ethnic minority older people by the year 2020.

To understand the nature of I&R services that are targeted to the aging, consideration must be given to the current and projected needs of our aging society. The explosive growth in the numbers and proportions of older people, especially, the oldest-old, will require that both public and private policies affecting health and long-term care, employment and retirement, housing and social services be considered with an aim to improve the quality of life of older persons. Fundamental issues will need to be resolved as to who will receive what resources and what will be the role of the private and public sectors in the care of older people. Ethnic minorities are

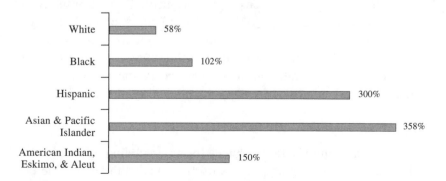

Figure 6.2 Population increase among ethnic minority older persons 65+ (1990 to 2020).

Source: "Administration on Aging: Planning for Longevity Across the Life Course."

expected to comprise nearly half of the U.S. population by the year 2050, a population growth fueled in part by increased immigrant and refugee populations. According to Torres-Gil (1992), it is anticipated that in many sections of the country a minority population will be a majority. Therefore, services to the aging minorities must be designed to accommodate the expanding older minority groups. The single female woman will predominate among the senior population, and it is estimated that more than 50% of women will be living alone. Older women in the future are predicted to remain significantly poorer than older men living alone. Though women will outlive their husbands by 15 years, on average they will earn only two-thirds of what their husbands had earned. Hence the plight of the single older woman will require special supports and community services (Hooyman & Kiyak, 1996).

This "Senior Boom" is impacting on our total society as "global aging" is occurring in many countries throughout the world, particularly in the nondeveloped countries. It is estimated that on average, one million people per month turn 60 around the globe, and the number of those 60 and over is projected to grow to 1.2 billion by 2025, with an increased proportion of older persons who are 80 and over (Stuen, 1999). These demographic data indicate that increases in longevity, expansion of the absolute number of older people, and diversity in the representation of ethnic minorities require that more accessible routes to information and needed services be considered.

Age is usually defined in chronological terms and is linked to life expectancy. With the lengthening of the life span, the term "aged" or "elderly" tends to be qualified with descriptive sequential categories such as "young old," "quite old," "very old," "old-old," and "the frail elderly." Irrespective of generalities, aging persons constitute a highly heterogeneous population. Hence, the aging process itself presents varying degrees of physical and mental limitations as well as social concerns that require individual help and assistance for support and quality of life.

REALITIES OF AGING: HARD CHOICES

In the provision of information services for an exploding aging population, the realities of the aging process itself also need to be considered. While normal aging does not lead to disability, the image of the helpless, disabled, and dependent aging person is gradually changing in favor of greater independence, health maintenance, and empowerment. A growing recognition of the creative capabilities and talents of older persons provides an effective defense against traditional ageism (Cohen, 2000). However, recognition must be given to the aging process itself, which inevitably involves individual physical and psychological changes. For example, changes in sensory functions, which include ability to see, hear, touch, taste, and smell, occur at different rates within the same individual and within the experience of groups of older adults. Bernice Hutchinson (1994) advises that "developing greater awareness of sensory changes associated with the aging process will increase the I&R provider's ability to offer positive support, promote independence, reinforce dignity, and improve service linkages." Because of the increased longevity of older persons, a greater number of older people will be living with chronic health conditions that will require information on choices in long-term care, including self-care and assisted living, and congregate care within local communities. Community care of older people is also required as increasing numbers of women, "the traditional caregivers," are employed outside the home.

In a changing climate of diversity, older adults and their caregivers face a complicated array of choices about their health care, pensions, insurance, housing, financial management, and long-term care. Hence there is an urgent need for access to local reliable information sources to assist seniors to arrive at informed personal choices. Since older people are living longer and are therefore faced with increased incidences of chronic illness and disabilities, personal home care services will be required in local communities to assist older adults who may be unable to rely on family care. What provisions in public financing of long-term care will be available? In view of disparities in health care, what choices in health services will be available under Medicare, Medicaid, and managed care? To what extent will the private sector support growing numbers of employees who have caregiving responsibilities for their elders? Will elder care be an important employee benefit in the next generation?

Housing for older persons requires an examination of individual needs, personal preferences, and availability and affordability of choices of housing. Though the proportion of older persons in nursing homes is as low as 5% at any one time, plans for long-term care include assisted living facilities, adult foster homes care, and availability of adult congregate homes. As more older persons live longer and healthier lives beyond the traditional retirement years, the need to provide a range of care options will continue to grow. A major problem in finding a suitable housing arrangement is often lack of information on the availability of housing choices to suit individual needs, preferences, and financial capabilities. Proximity to convenient access to shopping, affordable health care programs and availability of recreational activities will continue to be central concerns for effective community living.

New definitions of work and productivity present a phased work-retirement continuum for a population with a longer life span who will also have new opportunities for lifelong education and training. Though information technology provides a welcome opportunity to gain access to human services, how do we engage the older population in these benefits? This maze of choices demands an informed and empowered consumer as technology will continue to provide significant benefits in the lives of all older persons. How can we optimize the benefits of intergenerational programs that can be mutually helpful to both generations and strengthen the "ties that bind" (Kuhn, 1991)?

BENEFITS AND ENTITLEMENTS

The bulk of benefits and services for older adults has been provided by major legislative acts and programs that date back to the universal retirement benefits under the Social Security Act of 1935. Primary health insurance benefits have been provided by Medicare (on the federal level) and Medicaid (on a state level) since 1965. Of special significance to the field of I&R has been the OAA, originally enacted in 1965 and amended in 1973 to include mandated I&R services. Many of these legislated services require information on available choices, which present a confusing array of options and eligibility requirements that pertain to health care, housing, and long-term care. Following is a brief overview of some of the questions, dilemmas, and hard choices for which older persons require information, referrals, and assistance provided by a comprehensive resource system.

It is evident that the vast number of services that have evolved since 1935 and the subsequent changes in benefits and entitlements require knowledge of the rights, regulations, and limitations of the benefits involved. Given the current "ever-growing market basket of options" (Lambert, 1999), entitlements are often not known or understood, and therefore not acted upon. Changing benefits in public programs and an expansion of private sector services have contributed to the confusing consumer climate. Thus, older persons face a difficult array of choices that involve health care, housing, and financial management, as well as a selection of health insurance coverage, changing managed-care options, and limited coverage for prescription drugs. Needed guidance for management of retirement income is seriously lacking. How can one be helped to decide on options in retirement for continued employment as needed or desired? As for decisions on housing, older adults are often not familiar with the range of available senior housing or the conditions and requirements for subsidized housing. Even the distinction between universal Medicare insurance and the means-tested Medicaid program is often not clearly understood by aging persons, including those with marginal incomes who are unable to qualify for public programs yet are unable to pay for their prescription drugs and long-term care needs. While information on health services and health provisions are increasingly available on the Internet, the vast majority of older adults has limited access and insufficient familiarity with computerized operations to avail themselves of online data.

THE NATIONAL AGING NETWORK

THE PUBLIC SECTOR

In response to the watershed period of the 1960s and 1970s, which generated many social service programs on behalf of human rights and community services, it became apparent that the rapidly expanding older population was also in need of services located as close to their local communities as possible. Thus, Congress enacted the OAA in 1965 to be administered by the national AoA, which by 1973 established multilevel networks of federal, state, and local agencies. The major thrust of AoA was to plan and provide services to enable older persons to maintain their independence in their homes and communities. The OAA required that states and area agencies on aging shall "provide for the establishment and maintenance of I&R services in sufficient number to assure that all older individuals within the planning and service area covered by the plan will have reasonably convenient access to such services" (National Directory for Eldercare Information and Referral). To grasp the volume, range, and scope of existing information, referral, and assistance services for seniors, the Figures 6.3 and 6.4 graphically illustrate the available services for the aging in the public and private sectors, including profit and nonprofit agencies.

As seen in Figure 6.3, the National Aging Network, organized under the auspices of the U.S. Department of Health and Human Services, and operated by the AoA includes 57 State Offices on Aging at the state and territorial levels that are administered by NASUA. At the local level, 670 area agencies on aging are administered by the Association of the Area Agencies on Aging. The AoA also provides home and community-based services to 223 tribal organizations, which represent more than 300 American Indian tribes across the United States. Since the passage of the OAA in 1965, the aging network has developed a wide range of programs (see Figure 6.3) that literally serve millions of older consumers and their caregivers. The Information, Referral, and Assistance Programs designated as I&R/As are a basic service that also relate to the other major service programs, which include: Nutrition, the Long-Term Care Ombudsman Program, Case Management, Senior Centers, Legal Services, and Counseling for Pensions and Health Insurance.

Under the auspices of the AoA, the 1973 amendments to the OAA required that state and area agencies on aging "shall provide for the establishment and maintenance of I&R services in sufficient number to assure that all older individuals within the planning and service area covered by the plan will have reasonably convenient access to such services." As defined in the 1996–1997 directory, "Information and Referral/Assistance includes provision of information to individuals about public, voluntary, and private services or resources, and linkages to ensure that service will be delivered to the client." I&R/As also include contact with providers and caregivers in the interest of the older client. Often the first point of contact for assistance is the I&R/A service that receives the broadest range of inquiries relevant to the needs of older persons. According to a 1998 report on aging consumers (Vision 2000), I&R/As provide over 12 million contacts annually. It is estimated that the I&R/As also devote significant time and resources through outreach activities, which result in contact with an additional 1.5 million older persons during a given year. I&R/As receive the broad range of inquiries for older persons, which may involve simple information such as the location of a senior center, securing transportation, or the availability of literacy programs. On the other hand, I&R/As also respond to complex requests, which deal with housing options, eligibility for public benefits, referrals to assisted living facilities, and requests for crisis intervention.

Under the administration of AoA, three technologically related services

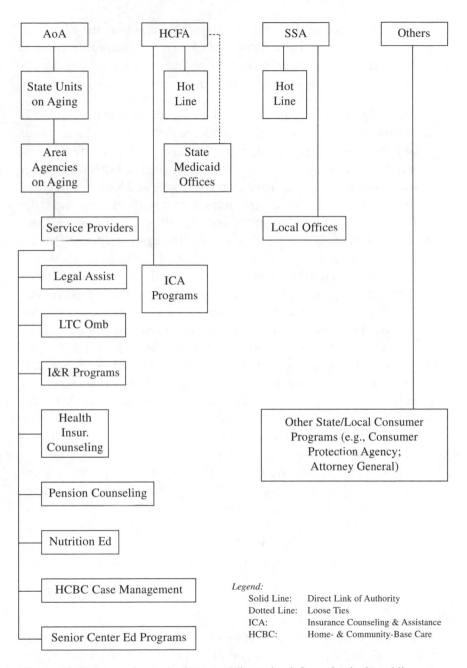

Figure 6.3 Universe of organizations providing aging information in the public sector.

Source: National I&R Support Center. *Vision 2000: Toward an Agency Information Resource System for the Next Century.*

have been developed in the field of aging, which include the Eldercare Locator, the National Aging Information Center, and the proliferation of AoA Web sites. All of these age-focused services rely on the capabilities of information technology.

1. The Eldercare Locator is a toll-free directory service (1-800-677-1116) that is designed to link the caller with the best available source of information on programs, resources, and services in the community where the older person resides. Established in 1991, the Locator maintains a database of more than 5,000 state and local providers of general and specialized information and assistance, such as the I&R/As, ombudsman programs, legal hot lines, and insurance counseling programs. Eldercare Locator is administered by NASUA and the local area agencies. The Locator reports an average of 6,200 calls a month and a cumulative total of 428,228 calls through March 1999. As might be expected, Home Health Aid receives the highest volume of calls. This toll-free service is designed to link the caller with the best source of information on programs, resources, and services in the community where the older person resides.

2. The National Aging Information Center is designed to provide data and share information on current approaches to practice and policy in regard to the aging. The collection of data on demography, health, and the social and economic status of older Americans is available at this website (http://www.aoa.gov) and is of interest to both consumers and providers of social services.

3. The directory of AoA Web sites offers the most comprehensive online national directory on aging. Through this organized directory consumers and their families have ready access to over 2,500 Internet informational sources. This national Web site also serves as an important link to the individual Web sites maintained by State Units on Aging and to approximately one third of the local Area Agencies on Aging.

THE PRIVATE SECTOR

As seen in Figure 6.4, information and referral services are provided by both nonprofit and for-profit organizations. In each of the nonprofit organizations, local affiliates are usually the direct service providers for aging information services. In the for-profit organizations, I&R services are incorporated as caregiver support services and may be included within Employee Assistance Programs that are provided by private corporations involved. In the public sector, hot lines are maintained by the Health Care Finance Administration (HCFA) and the Social Security Administration (SSA). In the private voluntary sector, a hot-line service is operated by the affiliates of the American Association of Retired Persons (AARP).

A *home health* industry for older persons has developed in the private sector. Since the early 1980s "care managers" have organized into a new group of caregivers, who are identified as private geriatric care managers. Rona Bartlestone, CSW, of Rona Bartlestone Associates in Fort Lauderdale, Florida, started the National Academy of Certified Care Managers in 1994 for the purpose of credentializing care managers. Families of geriatric clients are the major consumers of this private service (Cress, 1998). According to Ms. Bartlestone, "managers fill the role of families when parents are old, sick, and far" (*New York Times,* 1999).

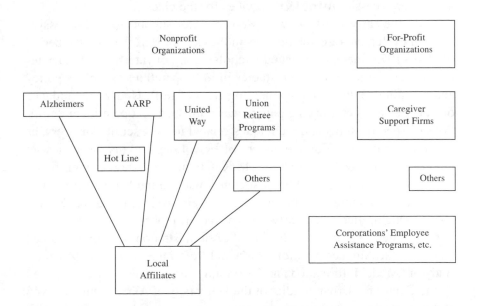

Figure 6.4 Universe of organizations providing aging information in the private sector.

Source: National I&R Support Center. *Vision 2000: Toward an Agency Information Resource System for the Next Century.*

PROMINENT ROLE OF THE U.S. ADMINISTRATION ON AGING IN I&R DEVELOPMENTS

In the relatively brief period of 40 years, during which I&R services evolved into a profession, the AoA has made a major contribution to this new field of professional practice through the support of research and training programs, interagency collaboration, and the application of information technology.

RESEARCH

The decade of the 1970s was a period of large-scale research projects that was sponsored by the AoA. In 1975 a study of applied management services, supported by AoA, reported the relative benefits and limitations of age-segregated versus age-integrated services. A general conclusion was that age-specific programs ultimately and inevitably also require access to generic age-integrated I&R services. Another extensive study sponsored by AoA was the three-volume evaluation of I&R services by Mark Battle & Associates, Inc. (AoA, 1977), which recommended greater availability and better accessibility of I&R services for the elderly.

Since the early 1970s, AoA has given major support to an impressive array of evaluative research projects in the field of I&R. During the period of 1970–1975, the AoA engaged Nicholas Long of Interstudy Associates to conduct a series of research studies in I&R operations as well as policy and planning analyses in the emerging field of I&R. Under the guidance of Long, a series of working papers was published on operational definitions of specific skills and techniques related to I&R service delivery, as discussed in chapter 2 on the history of I&R. Long and his associates set a precedent for I&R research and I&R networking. Another significant contribution that Long and his associates made to the beginning field of I&R was the annotated bibliography on I&R (Bolch, Long, & Dewey, 1972), which reflected an early state-of-the-art report.

Committed to I&R research, the U.S. Administration on Aging awarded a grant to the Alliance of Information and Referral Systems in 1981 for a study of "Model Information and Referral Systems." This study, conducted by the Center for Urban Studies at the University of Akron, Ohio, arrived at the selection of seven model systems. A major conclusion of this project was that I&R services are to be considered a *system*, which involves both public and private sectors (Shanahan, Gargan, & Apple, 1983).

AoA published instructional guidebooks on information and referral operations as early as 1975. A four-volume series of guidelines to establishing and maintaining I&R services included *Information and Referral: How-to Do It*. In 1977 a program development handbook entitled *I&R Services for the Elderly* was published for state and area agencies on aging and served as AoA guidelines for I&R service developments.

INTERORGANIZATIONAL PARTNERSHIPS

As discussed in the history of I&R (chap. 2), the AoA recognized the need for interagency networking in the operation of I&R services. As early as 1974, AoA established an Interdepartmental Task Force and entered into working agreements with other federal agencies and with representatives from private industry to promote I&R services for an aging population. Since 1992 AoA has participated in the annual training conferences conducted by AIRS and thereby has represented the special I&R interests of the older population. As of 1999, AoA has responded to the challenging problems of elder abuse by initiating collaborative service programs with other relevant organizations, such as HCFA and the National Center on Elder Abuse. AoA has also assumed the responsibility of training staff to assist older persons with Medicare + Choice programs, thereby informing older persons on their rights, benefits, and choices regarding Medicare entitlements.

IMPACT OF TECHNOLOGY ON AGING

Technology has the capacity to create "a virtual community" for aging persons. It provides opportunity for socialization, e-mail, listservs, and health information on the Internet. To promote greater mobility for body function, robotics is indispensable to promote independent living for increased numbers of older persons, who have varying degrees and types of incapacity. Advances in technology also serve remote rural areas through the application of computerization, and thereby bridge distances for older residents. Assistive devices can be extremely helpful for persons with a range of disabilities. Given the opportunity to provide patient care through technological communications, automated management of medical care can link patients with practitioners hundreds of miles apart. However, there are also serious constraints. Older adults may not have access to computers and may incur difficulties in operating automated devices due to limited vision, problems with arthritis, carpal tunnel, and the lack of necessary coordination. Therefore, while medical information on the Internet abounds, it may nevertheless serve only selected numbers of older adults.

Toward a National Strategy

The National I&R Support Center was established in 1991 as a concurrent strategy to the Eldercare Locator to enhance state, area agency, and local I&R system design and service delivery. The Support Center is also geared to assist aging I&Rs to meet the needs of a growing and diverse older population. As state and local area agencies instituted their individual programs, it became apparent that more regulation and consistency of I&R services were needed. In 1990 the National Association of State Units on Aging conducted a study, with AoA support, entitled "Toward a National Strategy to Enhance Information and Referral Systems for Older People." With the participation of focus groups to explore the role of I&R in assisting older persons, four major areas of concern emerged from this study, namely, inconsistencies in the quality of operations, deficiencies in personnel and staffing, problems in access to I&R, and lack of coordination among I&R systems. Based on the deliberations of these focus groups, standards for Older Americans Act I&R services were developed. These standards, which were published in September 1993, represented a milestone in I&R programming for older adult services. Concurrently, two supplementary publications were produced, which included an *Assessment Guide* and an *Implementation Guide for I&R Services* under OAA. These guides were regarded as valuable tools to promote visibility, improve access, and enhance I&R program development.

PARTNERING IN AN ERA OF I&R PROFESSIONALISM

In the year 2000, the AoA arrived at the decision to formally adopt and adapt the AIRS standards for professional practice in the field of aging. This represents a vital step in the universal adoption of the standards as published by AIRS and endorsed by UWA in 2000. Thereby, AoA has committed itself to the AIRS standards as a guide to quality practice in the aging network. A current consideration on *certification* has led to the decision to create an "Aging Specialty I&R Certification" program (*Information*, 2001) with a focus on professional service to the older consumer. To implement this program, the support center has organized an advisory committee to review relevant competencies for professional practice in the field of aging. Certification is projected for both staff working exclusively in the field of aging as well as for personnel engaged in services to older adults as well as other populations (National Aging I&R Support Center).

In addition to the phone operation of the national Eldercare Locator Service, AoA has also been an active partner in the design and implementation of the 211 nationwide telephone services. The endorsement of the *standards* and professional *certification* representing the three organizations within the I&R TRIAD reflect the strength of their partnership in achieving I&R professionalism.

SELECTED STATE INITIATIVES

A wide range of program initiatives are reported at the annual AIRS conferences that reflect the diversity of program developments in individual states. Following is a list of selected state initiatives that have been reported by various states as innovative programs for services to the aging:

1. *North Carolina:*   Division of Aging, which reported on policy papers and legislative priorities of aging advocacy groups, also a statewide directory of home and community care services.
2. *Alabama:*   planning of statewide 211 program, and the development of a statewide database.
3. *Hawaii:*   development of a single point of entry system for I&R services that will also be available at I&R kiosks.
4. *Illinois:* a kiosk system that includes general information on the entire human services system and collaborative efforts with private industry.
5. *North Dakota:*   a promotional effort that was launched with a recent PBS television special program called "Pulse on the Prairie," which was an opportunity to provide information on I&R programs to a large viewing audience.
6. *Tennessee:*   a discussion on planning for anticipated disaster services relevant to the aging population.

Other state initiatives that were also discussed on a teleconference peer exchange that aimed at a consensus-building process included enhanced use of technologies, updated training models, and more efficient staffing patterns. Within the public sector of services for the aging (as graphically shown in Figure 6.3) a wide variety of governmental agencies provide reports on various aspects of I&R services that operate at national, state, and local levels. Both HCFA and SSA conduct hot-line services. In addition to social security local offices, information on aging is also provided by state and local consumer programs such as the National Consumer Protection Agency and the state Attorney General's Office.

With the advent of a new millennium, various states have entered into studies of projected aging demographics and have suggested services for the older population within the individual state's future agenda. For example, the New York State Office for the Aging (1999 & 2000) developed a special initiative called "Project 2015." The basis of the projections for aging in New York is a report on demographic forecasts to the year 2025. This report depicts the changing ethnic composition of New York State and the rapidly growing 85-and-older age group. A similar study was conducted by the Minnesota Department of Human Services called "Baby Boomer Market Research Report" (1997). This study predicted that the population in 2030 will be more culturally and ethnically diverse; by 2050 older women will outnumber older men by two to one and older persons living alone will double by 2030. And although incomes will be higher than previous generations, there will be a growing disparity between the "have's" and "have-not's."

VISION 2010: A CALL TO ACTION PLAN

NASUA has projected the need for a seamless comprehensive aging information resource system for the 2000 century. In the proposed "A Call-to-Action" plan the aging network is assigned a strong leadership role in promoting I&R/A programs and in reaching the goal of a "comprehensive and coordinated system" that will "meet the needs of racially, culturally, ethnically, and geographically diverse groups of older consumers and their families." (Lambert, 1999). To achieve this goal, Lambert suggests a proactive approach to maximum communication, utilization of technology, responsiveness to older consumers and their families, and access to information needed for older consumers to make informed decisions.

CONCLUSIONS

This chapter focuses on the needs and challenges of a coordinated and comprehensive information and referral system in light of the current and projected burgeoning population of older adults. Despite the existing array of services and benefits for the aging in the public and private sectors, options and entitlements are often not known nor understood by older persons and their families. Based on an overview of the multilevel organizations that provide I&R services to the public, voluntary, and private sectors, a comprehensive information and resource system is promulgated for the aging. The role of technology is regarded as central to the development of shared databases that have the capacity to facilitate access to needed information and to provide new routes to human resources. The premise is that an informed older person has the capacity to be an empowered aging person, capable of self-help and informed choices. As adopted in the slogan of the International Year of the Aging 1999: "What is done for aging is done for all people." The I&R programs that have been developed in the field of aging have resulted in significant gains for the entire field of I&R. As successive cohorts of baby boomers enter into their senior years with far more mastery of information technology, they will be the senior "netizens" of the future. Given the expanded interest in information technology in the field of aging as well as in all human service fields, chapter 7 presents a discussion of selected models of I&R computerized systems.

REFERENCES

AoA. (1997). *Evaluation of information and referral services for the elderly: Final report*. Washington, DC: Mark Battle Associates.

Baby boomer market research report. (1997, June). *Aging Initiative: Project 2030*. Minnesota Department of Human Services.

Bartlestone, S. (1999, March 6). The growing business of helping the elderly to cope. *New York Times*, p. A1.

Bolch, E., Long, N., & Dewey, J. (1972). *Information and referral services: An annotated bibliography*. Minneapolis, MN: Institute for Interdisciplinary Studies.

Cohen, G. D. (2000). *The creative age: Awakening human potential in the second half of life*. New York: HarperCollins.

Cress, C. (1998). *GCM on the case: Case management moves into the geriatric age*. Cresscare. Case Management Agency for Elders. [online]. Avalable: http://www.cresscare.com; http://www.cresscare.com/articles/gcm_on_case.html.

Dychtwald, K., & Flower, J. (1989). *Age wave*. Los Angeles, CA: Jeremy P. Tarcher & Co.

Hooyman, N., & Kiyak, A. H. (1996). *Social gerontology: A multidisciplinary perspective*. Needham Heights, MA: Simon & Schuster.

Hutchinson, B. (1994). Bridging the gap: Enhancing communication with older adults. *Information and Referral: The Journal of the Alliance of Information and Referral Systems, 16*, 79–94.

Information and Referral Reporter, (1999, December). National Aging I&R Support Center.

Information and Referral Reporter (2001, July). National Aging I&R Support Center. Special Edition: Aging Specialty I&R: A Certification Program. Editor: Greg Case.

Kuhn, M. (1991). *No stone unturned.* New York: Ballantine.

Lambert, T. (1999). Vision 2010: Toward a comprehensive aging information resource system for the next century. *Information and Referral: The Journal of the Alliance of Information and Referral Systems, 21,* 105–119.

NASUA. (2000). *Certification for I&R specialists in aging: A white paper.* National Aging I&R Support Center.

New York State Office for the Aging. (1999 & 2000). *Project 2015: The future of aging in New York State. Articles and briefs for discussion & demographic projections to 2025.*

Profile of older Americans. (1998). *American Association of Retired Persons.* Washington, DC.

Shanahan, J. L., Gargan, J. J., & Apple, N. (1983). *Building model I&R systems: A bridge to the future.* Akron, OH: Alliance of Information and Referral Systems.

Stuen, C. (1999, Spring). User-friendly design. *Aging and Vision News, 1* (3), 1.

Torres-Gil, F. M. (1992). *The new aging: Politics and change in America.* New York: Auburn House.

Vision 2000: Toward a comprehensive aging information resource system for the next century. Washington, DC: National Association of State Units on Aging.

PART III

I&R Online

CHAPTER 7

Automating I&R Systems: Some Nuts/Some Bolts

Laura I. Zimmerman, PhD

INTRODUCTION

Technology has helped Information and Referral (I&R) specialists make great gains in the ability to perform their work. Whereas computers were rarely used for I&R prior to the late 1980s, it is rare that a computer is not used today. Unfortunately, there are still many, often rural, I&R programs that still do not have appropriate computer systems to support their work. This chapter attempts to give the I&R specialist information on some of the different models of I&R systems that are possible to use with today's technology as well as what to consider in setting up and improving I&R systems using available technology.

There are a number of different types of computer networks available today. An understanding of some basic terminology will be necessary to comprehend the technologies available for I&R systems. First, a *local* computer is the computer in front of you, either a laptop or desktop. It includes a keyboard and some type of display. In organizations in which there is a computer network, the database software for the I&R system may be on a different computer but can be accessed by the computer in front of you. Where the computer network is confined to a single building it is still usually considered *local*, and the network would be considered a *local area network* or a LAN. The defining factor in the ability for two or more computers to communicate with one another is the "protocol" or language that is used to communicate. On a LAN, a specific protocol is used to allow the computers to "talk" to each other.

The second most popular computer environment today for an I&R system is the Internet. The Internet is the network of networks around the world using a common communication protocol, Internet Protocol (IP), so these computers can "communicate" with one another. Each computer on the Internet has a unique IP address. Some computers (Web servers) have special software that makes them particularly useful for making data available for others to access. A number of I&R systems use the Internet in some capacity to collect or display their resource data. To do this a "Web server" must be used. A Web server is software that resides on a computer that allows it to "serve" information on the Internet.

There are other ways (protocols) of connecting computers beyond LANs and the Internet (i.e., mainframe computers). Since so few I&R systems use other protocols, this discussion will focus on LANs and the Internet.

At the least, Information and Referral systems consist of a basic list of community resources and information about these resources. The amount of data or number of resources in a system depends on a number of factors: (a) the focused area of the I&R, (b) the number of resources in the community, and (c) the size of the community or communities that the I&R includes. There are focused systems with just a few types of resources as well as more general statewide systems.

Regardless of size, for an I&R system to operate it must include some resource information. This information must be collected from the community resources included in the area and should be in some form useful to the I&R provider. Some organizations have notebooks or sticky notes on a board near the I&R provider's desk. These are the most basic of systems that use no searchable data system of any kind. More modern and larger systems have computer database systems; some are sufficiently sophisticated to easily share the resource data for use by other organizations. The most basic I&R will minimally have some resource data focused on the community population which it serves.

Some I&R systems also have a separate client database module. The data in this are gathered when a client contacts the I&R organization. The technologies used for the client database can be the same software or a completely separate system from that used for the resource data. The client data are often kept more confidential and available on a local computer or local network. Therefore, even though the same technologies can be used, the technologies for client data systems are often more secure. (In some organizations resource data are also kept secure in a password-protected environment on the Internet or on a LAN.)

There are a number of proprietary database systems in use by I&R organizations such as "Iris," "Refer," and "Tapestry," as well as a number of others. Each data system allows users to systematically search for resource data needed for their clients. Systems can also be developed from off-the-shelf database software such as Microsoft Access or FoxPro (these were actually used to develop Iris and Refer) or a number of other database systems. Whether the software system is I&R specific software or developed from off-the-shelf software for the user, the data have to be standardized and used in some sort of systematic format, as will be discussed later in the chapter.

I&R MODELS

There are three general models used for I&R systems. These models are based on the level of collaboration in the I&R "system." They range from those for individual organizations to those for large multicommunity and state systems. Prior to computer technology it was difficult to have multicommunity models that could access and share data and be kept up-to-date. Today, however, collaborative models are the norm, as organizations have banded together to reduce the costs of collecting and maintaining community data.

The simplest I&R model is also the oldest type. It is a totally "local" model or the individual I&R in which the data are collected and used by a single organization. Each individual organization may or may not use a searchable computer database. Some I&Rs, as mentioned previously, have all-paper systems, in which their data are not in a computerized form so it is not in an easily searchable format. Some have word-processed their inventory of community resources and therefore print and update a word-processed document. More sophisticated providers use a computer database system allowing the resources to be indexed in a number of different ways and therefore searched quickly using a computer. The major characteristic of this model is that the data are collected and used within the organization either on a single computer or a group of computers within a single organization. The computers can be networked or stand-alone, where each has a copy or some form of the software. Sometimes a manual is printed for those workers who are not as computer savvy (Zimmerman, 1991).

With the local in-house model, a single organization is responsible for obtaining and maintaining the entire system. This model is the most expensive to operate because the data collection and maintenance are all required of a single organization. The advantage to this system is that it meets the individual needs of the organization.

(SINGLE COLLECTION/MULTIPLE USE) MODEL

More and more shared systems are being incorporated due to the expense of maintaining I&R systems and the ability for the technology to allow it. After a systematic review of information systems in a North Carolina community, it was found that most human services organizations have some type of individual I&R model and were all collecting much of the same type of data. When the duplication was identified, it was recommended that the community services work together to develop single coordinated systems to reduce the costs of maintaining separate I&R systems. Shared systems are becoming more popular as service duplication is identified. The I&R software technology and Internet allow for greater sharing capacity within and among communities. These shared systems can range from two separate organizations to multicounty and statewide systems. Using systematic data collection efforts and similar software, attempts are being made to reduce the number of organizations collecting data and to increase the sharing of data from county to county (Zimmerman, 1999).

Shared data systems are probably the most popular model of I&R currently used. In this model a single organization collects, updates, and maintains the data for a number of organizations. The organization that maintains the data usually distributes the data in one of three formats, either through (a) an Internet site where a searchable copy of the resource data are available to anyone who wants to use it, (b) a searchable read-only version where other organizations can search a copy of the database on their local computer or computer network, or (c) on an exported copy of the data that an organization that has a copy of the I&R software can import for use. The second method is used when the organization has a separate client database for which client data may or may not be collected. The third distribution method is often used where the organization uses the client data-base module of the I&R software as well as the resource module.

With the use of this model, the responsibility for data collection and database maintenance does not necessarily need to reside in the I&R service organization. This responsibility can be handled by a separate organization or group within an organization that only handles data and data integrity as opposed to working with clients. This allows social work and other professionals to be freed up to work with clients and to worry less about data maintenance. However, the two groups do need to work together to ensure that appropriate data are collected and are valid for the system.

(MULTIPLE COLLECTION/MULTIPLE USE) MODEL

A third model that is not as popular but probably the most cost effective if coordinated and well organized is a multiple collection/multiple use collaborative. In this model, a group of organizations share in the data collection and data entry of a subset of data. The subset may be divided by service type (although these lines may not be clear) or by geographical area. Each organization then exports its specific data. It is then imported into a collaborative database and a single version is exported out of the collaborative data set for use by each unit. This model should be well organized so that data are not duplicated between units and the data are imported "cleanly" into the main database. This model allows for the sharing and responsibility for data collection and entry. These are typically the most time-consuming and difficult tasks for many organizations that maintain a large sharable system. A difficulty with this system is that many people have to learn how to enter the data in a standard format.

The problem of multiple people in different organizations entering data are alleviated with a variation of the second and third models, which divides the data collection task among many organizations. The organization that collects the data then gives it to a separate organization whose responsibility it is to enter and check the data in a single standard format. This takes some of the data collection burden off the data entry organization, but allows for greater consistency in the data entry.

Some advantages to the collaborative models, besides the reduction in cost of the data maintenance and updating, is that the data can be collected locally where providers have a good understanding of the resources. This is very important because unless there are reliable data, the system will not function optimally. Forms are sent to service providers to complete. Often the service providers who fill out the forms do not have a complete understanding of the I&R system and how the data are used. Therefore the data must be checked for accuracy and validity. Those who tend to refer clients and have knowledge of I&R are in the best position to perform this task.

In some communities such as El Paso, Texas, volunteers come together on a quarterly basis to review the data in the system and to discuss new resources or delinquent services (J. Windler & L. Sheldon, personal communication, 1994). Other communities, such as the Piedmont Triad region of North Carolina have local I&R providers obtain and review the information before passing it on to the data management organization (K. D. Berry, personal communication, 1999). A number of other models are used in other communities. What is important is that this task can meet the needs of the community and is performed locally.

With this task performed locally, and if the I&R software is the same and standardized across a number of communities, it is possible to create shared systems, where they are locally updated and exported for use in other communities. Technically, there is the ability to have a statewide system that is fed data from local units. The difficulty is in the coordination and standardization of such systems to meet the local needs and the larger needs for specific types of I&R and for more general I&R organizations. In North Carolina, the Aging Network is working toward such a model statewide (Zimmerman, 1999).

SETTING UP INFORMATION AND REFERRAL SYSTEMS

Setting up a new I&R system is a major project and cannot be considered as a light undertaking. The time it takes to set up a system using a searchable database is dependent on a number of varied factors. However, planning a new system with standard information, and then designing the system and inputting data are all vital in a strategic planning effort. Multi-organizational systems that have not been kept up-to-date or systems with no previous existence take approximately a year to set up and then another year to "get the kinks out." The following discussion focuses on a number of important aspects in setting up and maintaining an I&R system.

Any I&R system should be planned carefully, even for smaller systems in which only one person may be involved at the outset (or ever). Eventually, someone else will take over. Therefore, a good planning process will help document the system so everyone using the system will understand it. In larger community-based systems, it is important for as many users of the system as possible to be involved in the planning process. During the planning phase, a number of decisions must be made concerning the data that will be collected and how the I&R will operate. These include developing uniform data definitions, deciding how data will be obtained, and entering and checking the data. The data definition decisions should be made early in the process because the data must be decided upon *before* data can be collected. Once the collection process has begun, it is difficult to add additional data. For the specific operations of the I&R program, there is more room for adaptation and change even after the data system is in place.

There are a number of areas in which data must have uniform definitions to use within the database. The resource data include the agency data as one set of data and the service-program data, which can overlap or be a separate set of data, is a second set of data. A third set of data in the system includes key words and taxonomy data. The fourth set of data, if used, would be data on clients, and the uniformity of this data are dependent on how it will be used. There can also be other data in the I&R system that need to be defined and uniform, such as geographic area breakdowns, age breakdowns, and race-ethnicity distinctions. The need for these depends on the specific system, but should be standardized especially for multiorganizational systems.

The resource data for the agency, services-programs, and key words-taxonomy should be decided before the I&R specialist can begin to collect data for the system. For these areas it is best to decide what data are needed and to develop a skeleton of the database using the initial data fields. Once this is done, it is important to review this initial list and obtain consensus from those who will be using the system. This is a very important step. If this is not done carefully and prior to data collection, the needed data may not get into the system; consequently it is more difficult and costly to obtain data after the initial data collection step. Following the initial data collection, the most efficient way to obtain new data is during an annual update. These new data must be accentuated in the data collection process in order to obtain it with minimal follow-up.

The agency data usually includes data about demographics such as addresses, locations, phone numbers, types of services provided, World Wide Web (WWW) addresses, and e-mail addresses. This information is

especially important for larger agencies that provide more than one service. Depending on how the database is designed, it is possible to incorporate this section into the services-program data; however, this is not an
efficient way to set up the database nor is it advised. Instead, the agency
table should be related (linked) to the service-program data in a relational
type of database.

The service-program data are the data that are searched in the database.
There is typically more information needed in order to refer clients appropriately. It is important to make a decision on what data will be needed for
clients early in the planning phase. This is usually the first set of data discussed. This list of data can often be extensive so it is important to scrutinize the data that will be in this section. A balance is needed between
what data are useful for the different organizations using the system and
their clients, and what constitutes data overload. If an excessive amount
of data are included in this section, it may be difficult to obtain all the data
with accuracy. The large agency that may have 20 or more services may
have difficulty putting all this information together for the I&R program.
Again, it will be important to standardize definitions between programs in
which there may be different meanings of the same word, or different rules
pertaining to a set of data. It will also be important for someone to carefully review the data that are received from each agency. An organization
will often interpret the meaning of their services differently from how it is
used by the individual I&R specialist. This may occur as agencies try to
use the I&R as a free promotion of their services. It is difficult to overstate
the importance of clearly defining and *checking* the service data.

The key words used to search for the services-programs that fit client
needs also require careful attention from the onset. This is probably one
of the most problematic sets of data in the I&R system for a number of
reasons. First, personnel in the resource program that complete the data
forms usually do not have a good understanding of how key words are
used by the I&R specialist. Second, the personnel in the resource programs
often will have different definitions for what their service is from that of
the I&R specialist. These definitions not only change from agency to
agency, but also vary regionally. These two complications make matching
the key words to the services difficult. A third problem is deciding how
specific or general the list of key words should be. This is also somewhat
dependent on the amount of data in the system. A large metropolitan area
system, or a geographically expansive system that has a broad range of

services, would probably need more specific key words than a more rural I&R system.

A taxonomy of terms is sometimes used instead of key words, or key words are made up when I&R specialists are not familiar with how to use a searchable taxonomy (or a taxonomy incorporated into the software system). The Taxonomy of Human Services is the most popular taxonomy used in I&R. It is found in print form and has been incorporated into some I&R software in a logically defined hierarchy to enable the I&R specialist to search logical human service domains instead of key words. It tends to be more difficult to use than key words because of the lack of familiarity with the system, but once the specialist has gained familiarity, it is often more logical and preferred. The taxonomy has uniform definitions and is systematic which tends to fit well into the database concept (Sales, 1994).

Once the information that will be in the data system has been confirmed, the data then have to be collected. Data can be obtained in a number of different formats through a number of different methods. However it is collected, it should be done systematically. There are three basic methods for obtaining data using various technologies. All three methods fit data into a computerized database system. The differences involve the amount of human interaction used for each method. Before any data are collected, no matter the method, a letter should be sent out to the directors of the resource organizations explaining the system and the importance of obtaining the data for the system. Sometimes it is also helpful to obtain a letter from local community leaders to support the system and the data collection effort. A Public Service Announcement and a newspaper article can make the data collection effort more successful as well.

No matter which method is used, the order of the data is another important facet to the data collection effort. It is most efficient for the I&R specialist to obtain a clear understanding of how the data are entered into the system so that the data collection effort matches the order of the data as closely as possible. The specialist should enter sample data prior to developing the data collection forms to be familiar with the order of the data, as input into the software. If the data on the collection forms are ordered in the same sequence when entered, the data entry process will be much more efficient and less costly. The first method is a "paper collection system" in which forms with the needed data are sent to those community agencies that should be included in the database. The forms should be directed to a person, preferably the director of the agency or another I&R specialist, if the agency has one. Clear directions on how to complete the forms and return them should be included along with definitions for ambiguous data items. A phone number for questions should also be included. Including self-addressed stamped envelope is also helpful for increasing response rates. These forms can also be completed by phone, but this is more expensive and should be used as a follow-up by the specialist when the paper form is not received within a given amount of time. A reminder card should be sent out 2 weeks after the initial mailing if the data have not been received. The data is then entered into the computer system by the I&R specialist. The data need to be checked for completeness and accuracy, and this can be done prior to entering the data in the system or after the initial data entry.

The second method uses the worldwide web (WWW), a component of the Internet, as an interface to collect the data. In this method, an Internet form is designed to collect the data needed and someone then takes the data from the Internet database and puts it into the I&R database system. Examples include the Texas Statewide Information and Referral Network (http://www.hhsc. state.tx.us/tirn/tirnhome.htm), the Mid-East Commission Area Agency on Aging (http://www.mecaaa.org/), the Information and Referral Resource Network (http://www.ir-net.com/index.html), and Information and Referral of Vancouver, Washington (http://www.irccv. org/i&r/idx_i&r.htm). Some sites allow the forms to be downloaded and sent or faxed, in such as the Community Information and Referral of Central and Northern Arizona http://www.cirs.org/. The Internet is used as the interface, and a database can be used to capture the data, but for this method the data eventually end up in a different software system, usually in specialized I&R software.

Data entry into the I&R system is done by the specialist who also should carefully check the data for completeness and accuracy as well as judge the necessity of including it in the database itself. Since the WWW interface is open to anyone who goes to that location, it is important to differentiate among agencies that should have data in the system and those who should not. In general, community agencies are told about the Web site and asked to enter the data through the Internet using an Internet form instead of a paper form. This method is becoming more common as the Internet takes hold and as more people obtain Internet access and become more facile with the technology. Some advantages to this type of data entry system are that it can be faster and cheaper than mailing or faxing paper forms. The update can be performed anytime data changes occur, not only during the annual update. Also, a person can check the data. If set up correctly, this type of system could even facilitate quicker updating of data by allowing the service organizations to change only the data that need to be changed.

The third method incorporates the use of the Internet only, where data is entered directly into the I&R database system using an Internet interface. This method is generally used with closed systems (password protected), meaning that a person must have permission to enter the system, either to use it or make changes (by adding or changing their resource data) in the system. This is the most efficient system; however, one drawback is that there is no human in the process to check the data, which is an important step for having accurate data in the system.

Data entry must be done carefully and meticulously and should be checked thoroughly after it is done. Standards must be defined prior to beginning any data entry and some of these will be dependent on the software used. This includes capitalization and abbreviations. When working with computers and matching searches, the match may be dependent on exact capitalization so that "Senior Center" may not match "SENIOR CENTER" or "senior center." This is especially important if more than one person is entering data. If any special codes or abbreviations are used, they need to be standardized and entered the same way each time. Some systems have their own spell checks, but these will only catch words that do not have a dictionary spelling and not misspelled words that are still dictionary words.

The importance of the data-checking process cannot be overstated. When done properly, this is the most difficult part of the system. This part can be a real burden and lots of patience is required! The data must be carefully checked once it is entered both for data accuracy and for missing data. This is often better performed by more than one person and preferably not the person who enters the data. The system also needs to be checked to see whether it works the way it is expected to work. At this point there should be an assessment of the key words. If many services are found on a search, it may be necessary to use more specific terms for the key words to ensure the services are better differentiated. If a sufficient number of services are not found, then one needs to ask: Is the key word too specific? Are the services available in the community and simply missing from the database? Is there a gap in this area of service or is the I&R specialist unaware of the existence of the service? How important are the data to the system? Checking the data does not only mean to run a spell check. The data represent a system that must be assessed. Once the data have been collected and checked, the I&R specialist is ready to use the system, and if the data are to be shared, then this is the appropriate time for distribution of the relevant data.

DISTRIBUTIING DATA

Once the system is in place the distribution of data can be considered if there is a need to share the data. There are a number of options for distributing the data. These choices depend on the software used and the capabilities of those who use the data. There are many issues that need be resolved if the data are shared or publicly displayed. One major issue is the financial support that is raised for the shared system. Should data that are expensive to obtain be placed in a public environment for anyone to use without the ability to recoup some of the costs? Basically, many I&R organizations are not endowed with enough funds to adequately handle comprehensive I&R services. Therefore, consideration should be given for additional resources to support shared data. Another consideration is how will the data be used? Some human service providers feel there needs to be human intervention in the access to services and that the data may not be used appropriately. These are philosophic issues that may need to be discussed and resolved prior to making data public.

Data from the I&R system can be distributed in many ways. One of the oldest (and still useful) is through the use of a hard copy manual. Many human service providers like having the manual on the desk and are not yet accustomed to computerized formats. The printed manual is also easy to "sell" to recoup some of the costs of collecting the data, putting the manual together, and getting it distributed. The manual, however, does not allow for some of the functionality of a computerized version. Another downside to the printed manual is that it is quickly outdated, often before it gets into print. For those who use a computer version, it is always possible for a user to print out the latest data from that computerized version, thus having a more current print version.

Some I&R software packages allow the searchable database to be distributed to other computers. Read-only data versions allow for a completely searchable system without a client database or the ability for changes to be made to the system. Some I&R software allows the database to be exported into another copy of the same software, thus allowing the I&R specialist to maintain the data and then be able to share it with other organizations on a regular basis. These methods allow the responsibility for maintaining the data system to be held by one organization while many organizations can reap the benefits.

A third method for distributing data from a local I&R database includes the use of the Internet. Some I&R software packages allow the program data to be exported into a crude, Internet-compatible form. This method is becoming more popular. A savvy database and web programmer can also manipulate the exported data to make an "easy-to-use" interface for the system. The more intricate these web systems become, the more functionality they have; however, they are more expensive. Some examples of online data systems can be found linked to http://ssw.unc.edu/hssa/maps/maps.html.

Some software programmers have developed Internet-only I&R data systems, which display only through the Internet. Most of the systems that are totally Internet-based are private systems that are password-protected, allowing only those involved with the system to access it. However, as the Internet becomes easier to use, more reliable, and faster, there will probably be more I&R systems that will be only available through the Internet.

TRAINING USERS

Training is important for those who will be using the I&R data system. Typically, there are orientations or orientation manuals for newly hired employees. There should be similar manuals for users of an I&R system. This manual should cover how the software works (often there is an available software manual). The manual should also include standards used in the particular system for data collection and data entry, as well as standards for checking the data and other particulars of the system.

Since many I&R database systems are complex, there may also be the need for more formalized training, especially for an implementation of a new system. There are a number of methods for training new system users including one-on-one, videotape, computer training modules (if available), lecture, and hands-on training. Hands-on training tends to be the fastest way to get new users up to speed. I&R users can practice on the system and be able ask an instructor questions about the system. Training should be timely, done in small groups, and based on a sample of the data system they will be using. Timely means that training should occur as close to the time a new systems comes into use as possible. Ideally, a worker should return from training and immediately be allowed to use the live system or a practice system. Often training takes place long before a computer system is available for use, and then the effects of training are lost. After using the system for a while, videotapes and other less expensive training methods are useful for increasing skills when the trainee is ready for more material. Training in other skills such as answering a phone and listening to clients is also necessary, when indicated. All these skills are vital to the success of an I&R system.

UPDATING THE SYSTEM

Updating the I&R data system is probably the most important task and responsibility of the I&R specialist. Failure to update the data decreases the usefulness of the system and frequently leads to the failure of many I&R systems. The use of technology can make it easier for updating to be performed on a more regular basis.

Prior to the use of computer technology, I&R system updating was usually performed at least annually. A copy of the system's current data would be sent to the agencies and the agencies were asked to send back changes. This was, and is, still done on a variety of time schedules. Some organizations prefer to do this once a year, every 6 months, or even more often; others are updating different data groups continuously, that is, certain letters of the alphabet each month.

This system works well for agencies already included in the I&R system, but it is also important to have "feelers" out for new agencies that may not be in the database. Some organizations do this by having a voluntary meeting for the specialists from the various human service groups. They might meet annually to discuss the system and consider additional services or any other needed changes. This type of meeting allows system users in the same specialty area to communicate and share input about the system to the I&R specialist.

Internet technology can further facilitate the updating process. Using data entry processes based on the WWW allows data to be updated whenever there are changes and not only during annual updates. As more and more human service providers gain access to the Internet, this method of updating is becoming more viable. The speed and timeliness of this method allow for seasonal changes in the database or funding changes. Depending on other technologies used in the I&R system, it is technically possible to make these changes available quickly to others using the system (even in a matter of minutes or hours).

As discussed previously, it is possible to have the data entered directly into an online system with no human interaction; however, the preferred process is for the data to come in and then have changes and additions entered manually into the I&R system. This second method allows for a data validation step, which always improves the system.

ANALYSIS AND REPORTING

There are many opportunities for analyzing data and reporting information from an I&R database system. Technically, any database field can be analyzed for frequencies, or it can be related to any other variable. Many I&R database systems have reporting systems built in as well as a build-your-own report module. These may not always look attractive for a finished report, but a savvy I&R specialist who understands the data can easily make it presentable by using software programs such as Excel and PowerPoint.

The type of data needed depends on its use. If community coordination is favorable, then an I&R database system can allow for sophisticated analysis. For example, it is theoretically possible to obtain unmet needs data across the community if all human service organizations collect the information. The analysis and reporting are usually a function of the ability of an I&R specialist to envision outcomes from the data and apply a knowledge of statistics to data analysis. This is an area that may be very useful to investigate because reports based on reliable data from the system may help make a good case for additional funding. Well-organized data can also aid an agency in proving organizational effectiveness.

CONCLUSIONS

Computer technology has changed our society in a number of ways. It has facilitated the ability for I&R specialists to provide access to services for a community. Prior to the use of computer technology, it was difficult for I&R systems to be designed for anything beyond one local unit. Now the use of technology allows many opportunities for collaboration in designing community and intercommunity systems. It is now possible for many organizations to be involved in the development, data collection, and even data entry of a system that they will be operating. Instead of purchasing a hard copy manual of resource services, which may or may not meet their particular clients' needs (and may even be outdated), agency staff will have immediate access to computerized data that can be sorted and selected in many useful ways.

Specialized I&R software also allows for a more comprehensive data list, which in turn can incorporate the needs of many organizations simultaneously. The database is quickly searchable and the appropriate data can be printed for the client as indicated. Further, these systems frequently allow the collection of client data for service providers to improve their services to clients. The availability of computerized databases has brought about extraordinary changes in I&R services which, in turn, has allowed easier access to human services. The challenge now is to inform all citizens of the availability of such information systems and ensure that they get access to the appropriate system when needed. With electronically organized data, agency staff have the capability to gather information on usage and report gaps in service areas (e.g., clients' unmet needs).

Dedication: This chapter is dedicated to the memory of Marti Pryor Cooke, Director of Social Services, Orange County, North Carolina, 1988–2000. Through Marti's perseverance to have a better and more coordinated information system in Orange County, she involved me in an evaluation of information in all the human services in 1990. This led to the need for a coordinated Information and Referral system in Orange County. I later worked with Orange County United Way to assess software and implement an I&R system. This system is now a multicounty system operated by the Triangle United Way. This was the first of seven I&R systems that I have helped communities and organizations plan and implement.

REFERENCES

Zimmerman, L. I. (1991). *An assessment for the human services management team's master client index file, Orange County, N.C.* (Technical Report). Human Services Research and Design Laboratory, University of North Carolina at Chapel Hill.

Zimmerman, L. (1999). *Information and assistance: Meeting the needs of the aging population in the new millenium.* Chapel Hill, NC: Human Services Smart Agency, University of North Carolina at Chapel Hill.

Sales, G. (1994). *A taxonomy of human services.* Los Angeles, CA: The Information and Referral Federation of Los Angeles County, Inc. and the Alliance of Information and Referral Systems.

SUGGESTED READINGS

Alliance for Information and Referral Systems Newsletter. Published by Alliance for Information and Referral, Seattle, Washington.

Childers, Thomas, (1984). *Information and Referral: Public Libraries*. Westport, CT: Greenwood Publishing Group, Incorporated, ISBN: 089391147X.

Hawley, George S. (1987). *Referral Process in Libraries: A Characterization and an Exploration of Related Factors*. Lanham, MD: Scarecrow Press, Inc. ISBN: 0810820102.

Levinson, Risha W. (1987). *Information and Referral Networks: Doorways to Human Services*. New York: Springer Publishing Company, ISBN: 0826148204

Zimmerman, L. I., & Bowen, N. K. (1999). Rural information and referral services: Serving North Carolina's elderly population. In I. Carlton-LaNey, R. L. Edwards, & P. N. Reid (Eds.), *Preserving and strengthening small towns and rural communities*. Washington, D.C.: NASW Press.

Zimmerman, L. (1999). *Information and Assistance: Meeting the Needs of the Aging Population in the New Millenium*. Chapel Hill, NC: Human Services Smart Agency, University of North Carolina at Chapel Hill.

Zimmerman, L. I. (1997). Information and referral: A closer look at one software package. *Smart Bytes, 3* (3), 1, 3.

Zimmerman, L. I., & Broughton, A. (1996). Information and referral systems for human services. *Smart Bytes, 2* (3), 3.

CHAPTER 8

Staffing and Training for "High Touch/High Tech"

*The staff of the (I&R) service shall be composed of
competent, ethical, qualified individuals, sufficient in
number to implement the policies of the service.*
Corazon Estava Doyle, 1974.

C ontrary to the familiar phrase that denotes "high tech/high touch,"
the order of these two components has been reversed in the title of
this chapter to emphasize that the "human touch is the primary task,
and the high tech component is a means to optimize the human services."
To date there is no prescribed nor ideal model for the staffing of I&R programs. Given the multiplicity of agencies and the myriad entries to services, the responsibility of meeting the service needs of all citizens appears
overwhelming. What constitutes an adequate or optimal number of personnel? What training or educational qualifications are required? What
variables need to be taken into account to arrive at an estimate of adequate
staffing? A review of existing staff levels in I&R agencies reveals marked
differences and reflects a unique mix of volunteers, paraprofessionals, and
professionals. As professional I&R standards have been published and as
formal requirements for certification have been established with specifications for the Certified Information and Referral Specialist (CIRS) and
the Certified Resource Specialist (CRS), a new professionalism in I&R
staffing has evolved. The rapid expansion of information technology has
also added a new dimension in staffing and training for I&R operations,
as shown in the CIRS model in Table 8.1.

MULTILEVEL STAFFING

Staffing patterns vary enormously in I&R agencies. Some I&R services may be provided by a single staff person, while other agencies may operate with extensive staff involved in million dollar budgets. As diminishing numbers of I&R programs rely on the "shoe box file," a growing number of agencies depend on staff that can operate or are capable of learning to operate computerized systems. Some I&R agencies operate totally with a professional staff, while other I&R programs are staffed predominantly by volunteers. I&R service programs that are operated by multiple levels of staff including professionals, paraprofessionals, and volunteers have different backgrounds, varied experiences, and individual levels of expertise. Job descriptions tend to vary in accordance with the organizational mandate for various levels of staff. With the advent of the antipoverty programs in local communities in the 1960s, I&R services were primarily staffed by paraprofessionals and volunteers. The predominant pattern of I&R staffing currently reflects multilevel personnel who combine the talents and skills of professionals, paraprofessionals, and volunteers in varying proportions.

VOLUNTEERS

Volunteers may constitute the largest number of I&R agency staff. The role of the volunteer is particularly dominant in local I&R organizations that are associated with local community programs, hot lines, and services to older people. Special interest groups including women groups, labor unions, and various health programs dealing with I&R relevant to specific disorders such as cancer, heart disease, and stroke are heavily staffed by volunteers. National organizations such as the Volunteers of America, the Voluntary Action Centers, and the American Red Cross rely primarily on the trained volunteer to staff their I&R-related programs. Because volunteers are often acquainted with informal resources as well as formal services, and are generally knowledgeable about the local mores, norms, and sociocultural traditions of the local community, volunteer staff can significantly enhance effective I&R delivery.

The stark realities of shrinking budgets and staff cutbacks that have occurred intermittently since the early 1980s have tended to generate increased volunteer staffing. However, the recruitment and retention of volunteers are not without problems. The availability of the traditional volunteer homemaker is rapidly diminishing, as larger numbers of women are joining the workforce. Volunteers are increasingly sought from the ranks of older citizens, particularly the retired elderly who wish to remain active in community services. The continued expansion of the Retired Senior Volunteer Program, a federal volunteer program, provides a growing pool of older volunteers. Other sources for I&R volunteers are persons interested in a potential career in community services, including students in preprofessional training in the helping professions (e.g., social work, librarianship, nursing, teaching, and other human relations disciplines).

A notable example of a national organization staffed by 85–90% volunteers is the network of British Citizens Advice Bureaus (CABs). Volunteers are required to complete a mandatory training program to prepare primarily for direct services in local CAB programs. The required training course for CAB volunteers is monitored by the central office of the National Association of Citizens Advice Bureaus (NACAB), which provides training materials and consultants to ensure "quality" training programs. One of the unique features of the CAB is the volunteer solicitor, who is available on *a rota* basis for legal counsel to I&R clients by scheduled appointment. Town planners and accountants are also called upon to volunteer their services at the request of a CAB worker. The availability of legal counsel due to the no-fee policy of the British solicitor may also explain why CAB programs tend to assume a stronger consumer advocacy role than is generally found in American I&R programs. It is generally agreed that the volunteer can succeed only to the extent that adequate and competent supervision is provided.

PARAPROFESSIONALS

Paraprofessionals constitute a significantly high proportion of I&R personnel, many of whom are also involved in administration and community organization as well as direct client services. For many paraprofessionals an I&R experience can serve as a career ladder and as an incentive to qualify for the CIRS designation. For other paraprofessionals, I&R can provide a full-time career, even without formal academic credentials. Encouraged by the expansion of consumer participation in community service agencies, a corps of paraprofessionals evolved in the I&R programs of the 1960s with varying levels of education and diverse backgrounds. Much of the success of the local community action programs of the early 1960s depended upon paraprofessional staff who were aware of service barriers and who brought to I&R programs a unique and intimate knowledge of the local community and its residents. The dual consumer-provider roles of paraprofessionals tend to provide firsthand information on the existing problems in the community and knowledge of informal routes in gaining entry to local services.

Paraprofessionals have also been referred to as "indigenous personnel," thereby denoting neighborhood residents who work in local community I&R programs. It has been suggested that indigenous personnel have an advantage over professional workers in their ability to communicate more effectively with the disadvantaged groups in the community, particularly with the economically depressed. It has also been argued that indigenous personnel gain greater trust from clientele and are apt to be more partisan than their professional counterparts. Kahn (1966) rejected this allegation, insisting that "an indigenous identity has as many special pressures and built-in limitations affecting performance as a professional identity, without as many checks and balances." While budgetary constraints may be a major reason for hiring volunteers and paraprofessionals rather than professionals, the critical issue in differential staffing is the competence and effectiveness of the I&R service performed by each level of staff is in accordance with appropriately delineated tasks. The opportunity for I&R personnel to gain certification as CIRS staff has since 1997 added a new and well-recognized level of professional attainment.

PROFESSIONALS

The quest for professional status for I&R agents and from other human service disciplines has involved two sets of I&R professional staff: (a) the service professionals who seek to utilize I&R services in their own professional practice (e.g., social workers, nurses, librarians and teachers), and (b) the CIRS and the CRS, both of whom are in I&R practice. Thanks to the development of the AIRS Certification Program, I&R staff members can now qualify to become CIRSs or CRSs and thereby gain professional status and recognition. A new certification program for CRSs was launched by AIRS in 2000. The application process is the same as for CIRS but the examination covers the following resource specialist competencies (Cueny & Sales, 2000):

1. General knowledge and skills,
2. Demonstrated resource database maintenance skills and abilities, and
3. Work-related attitudes for resource specialists.

Since the mid-1960s, a wide variety of health and social service professionals have become involved in I&R programs that operate in various settings including libraries, schools, hospitals, military installations, and a wide array of other health and social service agencies. By the early 1970s, librarians began to create I&R programs such as the TIP program in Detroit and the LINK program in Tennessee, which originated as an interdisciplinary program conducted by a librarian and a social worker. An early survey of I&R multidisciplinary training programs conducted by AIRS in colleges and universities in 1983 revealed significant numbers of I&R training programs conducted at Schools of Medicine, Nursing, Public Health, Library Science, and the behavioral sciences. This survey was conducted by Anne C. Goldenberg, chair of the AIRS Professional Training and Education Committee, who stated that "the purpose of this committee was to integrate the body of knowledge of I&R practice into the curricula of colleges and universities." The main objective of this effort was to survey existing I&R courses and I&R programs with a view toward promoting model courses and programs at professional schools in coordination with AIRS and United Way of America. An added objective was to promote research in international access programs, such as the British CAB. While the results of this survey were reported at successive AIRS conferences (1983–1987), the effort was short-lived but nevertheless of interest in its far-reaching perspective (Goldenberg, 1986).

Prior to I&R certification, the broadly defined tasks of I&R service delivery led some professionals to dismiss I&R "as a given," assuming that I&R is an inherent responsibility of all helping disciplines. Moreover, some professionals have been prone to regard I&R services as less than a professional responsibility and therefore relegated I&R tasks to lower levels of nonprofessional staff and volunteers. Another constraint was that some human service professionals tended to view the new application of information technology in I&R operations with some misgivings. One objection was that automated responses to client requests may result in alienation between workers and clients. Another long-standing argument was that professional confidentiality may be threatened by computer operations. The fact that professionals, as I&R providers, have often not been accorded due recognition in status, salary, or career advancement may also have contributed to the reluctance of some professionals to recognize I&R as a professional service.

Although human service professionals are aware of the persistent problems in gaining access to needed services, some professionals still appear to be reluctant to grasp the significance of utilizing organized access systems and shared databases. Even Nick Long, a psychologist and a distinguished pioneer researcher in I&R programs during the early 1970s, questioned whether professionals should be involved in I&R operations and, if so, in what capacity. His conclusion was that professionals should not be direct service agents but should restrict their activities to the tasks of administration, training, planning, and research (Long, 1974). Assuming a broader stance, Kahn (1966) maintained that I&R services should be "professionally directed" and that professionals should provide guidance and supervision to paraprofessionals and volunteers, however, not to the exclusion of assuming a role in direct client services. Other professional authorities have also acknowledged the importance of facilitating access to resources and services, but have questioned whether I&R services add an additional bureaucratic layer to the already complex structure of professional service agencies (Gilbert and Specht, 1974). The above-alleged complaints are losing cogency as information technology is continuing to demonstrate its relevance and effectiveness in information and referral operations. Given the combined application of information technology and professional helping skills, I&R is forging new routes to human services.

INTERDISCIPLINARY I&R PROGRAMS

Recognizing that I&R provision is not the domain of any single discipline, efforts are being made by professionals to engage in interdisciplinary partnerships, which tend to reduce professional competitiveness by developing complementary relationships among professionals. Greater appreciation of the particular skills of "professionals by professionals" has demonstrated the value of tapping the specific competencies of I&R-related disciplines. For example, the report of the I&R Task Force of the National Commission on Library and Information Science (National, 1983) strongly recommended that the human relations skills of the social worker can effectively complement the informational expertise of the librarian.

Under a federal grant from the Administration on Aging (AoA), awarded to the Adelphi University School of Social Work in 1984 (Grant No.

90AT0126), social work interns from the Adelphi School of Social Work and library interns from the Palmer School of Library and Information Science (Long Island University, CW Post Campus) participated in the interdisciplinary I&R training project known as Senior Connections. The thrust of this project was to enable students from both professional schools to develop I&R services in selected local public libraries with the participation of older volunteers. Following the initial grant from the AoA in 1985, annual funding from the New York State legislature expanded this program to additional libraries under the overall administration of a professional social worker. While the interdisciplinary student training program was discontinued in 1995 when the program was transferred from the Adelphi School of Social Work to the Nassau County library system, the trained older volunteers, as I&R agents in public libraries, have continued to expand I&R services in public libraries (Levinson, 1996).

The cross-disciplinary nature of I&R, which extends beyond the institutional boundaries of service agencies, involves complementarities of functions and a recognition of the benefits of interdisciplinary relationships. For example, in assuming the I&R role, librarians have become aware of the junctures at which a social worker with personal helping skills and community organizational experience can contribute to a more comprehensive I&R service, particularly in the development of interagency relationships, problem delineation, referral methods, and the application of the professional helping relationship. Likewise, social workers have come to appreciate the informational and technical skills of the librarian and the opportunities for client entry and re-entry via a public library-based I&R service. The library is a local community center to which a client-patron can turn to and return to as circumstance or change of condition may warrant. Similarly, librarians have come to realize that the social worker can follow up and retain accountability for services to the patron-client at various junctures in the helping process at which the librarian may elect or be constrained to continue contact. On the other hand, librarians are trained information specialists who have made significant contributions to the emerging field of professional I&R as practitioners, as authors of many articles in the AIRS journal, and as researchers in information systems and evaluation.

Significant gains in planning and research have also been achieved by professionals by sharing of a common database of community resources. The database presents an excellent opportunity for cross-professional pooling of information in assessing community needs, service gaps, and inadequacies, as well as in projecting plans to reach the unserved and the potential consumer. The complementary relationship that has been demonstrated between social workers and librarians in the Senior Connections training program is also applicable to partnerships that involve other professionals in I&R service delivery including nurses, teachers, counselors, therapists, and other helping professionals (Hezel & Jacobson, 1987).

It is possible, nevertheless, to recognize that professional resistance and bias can exist and seriously hamper professional collaboration. For example, librarians may be reluctant to pursue complex patron problems lest they cross professional lines into the social workers' domain of diagnostic casework and treatment. Moreover, librarians have at times seriously questioned the appropriateness of the advocacy function in library-based I&R service delivery, asserting that advocacy may conflict with the neutrality of traditional library services (Gaines, 1980; Kopecky, 1972). Furthermore, handling personal identifying information in the referral process may be regarded by the professional librarian as inappropriate and intrusive. It is interesting to note, however, that Childers negated this alleged negativism and confidently suggested that "the great scepter of 'social work' may be imaginary and that experience may cause it to evaporate" (Childers, 1984).

Similarly, social workers have also adhered to their own professional biases and have questioned whether the public library is an appropriate setting for personal helping services, particularly since libraries have been traditionally regarded as middle-class institutions that serve only the literate reading public in a "hush-hush atmosphere," an impression that libraries have long dispelled. Whatever reluctance exists on the part of professionals may be significantly overcome by a clearer understanding of the respective service roles involved in I&R provision, and a sharing of the capabilities of information technology and common databases.

THE CERTIFIED I&R SPECIALIST (CIRS): A ROLE-TASK ANALYSIS

The professional role of the I&R provider was generally undefined until the mid-1990's. With the support and guidance of the AIRS board of directors, certification of I&R staff was created in 1996. Certification represents the legal control of the use of the title of CIRS. As all "helping professionals," I&R providers share important professional characteristics such as specialized knowledge and skills, a code of ethics, self-regulation, and membership in their own association or alliance (Frederico, 1990). The AIRS (1996) CIRS Application Packet specifies the competencies that an I&R specialist is required to demonstrate in carrying out job-related responsibilities. Individuals that meet the eligibility requirements may submit an application, which, if approved by AIRS, permits the candidate to take the scheduled examination. Successful candidates who pass the AIRS certification examination are entitled to use the designation of CIRS after their names.

Peter Drucker, a well-known authority in organizational management, offers some fresh insights into management in the information age. Drucker (1995) advises that information specialists should be "data literate; know what to know." He asserts that "a database, no matter how copious, is not information; it is information ore, and information specialists are the tool makers." Another applicable concept to I&R management is Drucker's assertion that "knowledge workers work in teams and are of necessity specialists within given organizations."

Table 8.1 suggests that the roles and tasks of the CIRS, are not mutually exclusive nor does one area of expertise supercede the other. As noted on the table, the CIRS professional is involved in a variety of roles, including direct services to clients, participation in the management of the organization, and the application of appropriate levels of information technology. Following is a discussion of each of the specializations of the CIRS.

THE HUMAN SERVICES SPECIALIST

In the area of human services, the CIRS is a direct service intermediary who offers brief or extended I&R Services, as may be indicated. For cases in which the client is unable to mobilize or follow through on a plan for needed assistance, the I&R specialist may take on the role of the case advocate by acting on behalf of the person or the family in need of help. In providing direct services to the client, the I&R specialist is held accountable for the interview and referral, as indicated. The maintenance of updated information and systematically organized databases (resource files) is imperative. Helping the client formulate a plan or arrive at a course of action are desired goals. The I&R task may involve brief counseling or referral to another agency, based on an appropriate professional diagnostic assessment. If the need for extended counseling is indicated, the serv-

TABLE 8.1 The Certified I&R Specialist (CIRS)—A Role-Task Analysis

Specialization	Roles	Tasks
I **Human Services Specialist (client-focused)**	Service intermediary	Brief term I&R services Extended I&R services
	Case advocate	I&R services on behalf of client
	Crisis intervention agent	I&R specialist response to individual, family, and community crises / emergencies.
II **Organizational/ Management Specialist (agency-focused)**	Policy advocate/ administrator	Social policy/social action Intra-agency management Networking-interagency linkages Outreach/public relations
	Systems analysis/ evaluator	Data analysis Service effectiveness Service efficiency Service evaluation—outcome analysis
	Educator/trainer	Staff development and training Staff supervision
III **Information Technology Specialist (systems-focused)**	Researcher/systems designer	Profiling agency operation Feasibility study Consulting with board and staff Involving appropriate consultant
	Analyst/planner	Setting objectives Choices of hardware and software Determining costs
	Systems operator	Implementing the database Developing a user manual for staff Training and testing Modifying information Technology system

ice intermediary may provide a more intensive level of counseling or refer the client to an appropriate resource. Selective or universal follow-up will depend upon agency policy and the provider's judgment of the client's readiness and capacity to follow up on a referral. Should the client be unable to follow through on the given information or the indicated course of action, the I&R agent may then assume the role of the case advocate on behalf of the individual client or clients involved.

Because of the ability of I&R services to respond to requests for assistance with immediacy, the CIRS professional is prepared to apply crisis intervention in the event of natural disasters such as floods, hurricanes, tornadoes, and earthquakes. Crisis intervention is also applicable to personal crises such as divorce, drug abuse, and suicide.

THE ORGANIZATIONAL-MANAGEMENT SPECIALIST

In assuming the role of the Organizational-Management Specialist, the CIRS administrator is responsible for intra-agency management of the I&R agency as well as for developing and maintaining linkages with other relevant organizations on an interagency basis. In the category of indirect services, the class or policy advocate may undertake action on behalf of aggregates of clients who have reported a common problem or concern. For example, Detroit residents elected to raise their property tax to restore the hours of service in local public libraries as a result of a vigorous "Keep the Doors Open" campaign. Users of the library-based I&R services were organized and were among the staunchest supporters of the protest (AIRS, 1984).

A key role in I&R operations is assumed by the administrator, who carries out the major responsibilities of hiring personnel and delineating staff assignments. Other vital administrative responsibilities include the sharing of program priorities and the implementation of organizational decisions related to staff operations and agency budgets. The role of planner-researcher is an administrative task that entails agency planning and agency evaluation in testing service effectiveness and agency efficiency. The extent to which planning and research can be carried out will depend upon agency policy, available resources, and the commitment and readiness of the administrator and agency staff to engage in the planning-research process.

The educator-trainer role entails tasks for educational and training programs to enable staff to carry out the service delivery program and to operate the existing level of information technology. I&R agencies may have in-house staff with the background, experience, and capability to conduct training programs. However, if staff trainers are not available within the agency, outside consultants may be hired to provide the advice and expertise required for staff training. Essentially, I&R training is a continuous process that needs to be provided for all levels of staff in accordance with their respective responsibilities and essential tasks.

THE INFORMATION TECHNOLOGY SPECIALIST

To carry out the responsibility of initiating and maintaining an information technology system, it may be advisable to engage a professional consultant who can guide the process of establishing and operating an information system. The expense of hiring a consultant may be well rewarded as to investment of time, costs, purchase of appropriate hardware and software, and staff training. It is helpful to engage a consultant who can "take the mystery out of" complex concepts and unknown terminology to staff. It is vital to enhance communication between human service professionals and technically oriented systems designers to arrive at sound decisions for hardware and software applications. Though I&R consultants may be called upon at any time in I&R agency operations, the guidance and advice of a consultant can be especially helpful in modifying or instituting a *new* information system.

Manikowski (1990) advises that introducing a computer into an agency can greatly enhance and facilitate the operations that staff can perform. In fact, he asserts that "the horizons of your automated system will be limited only by your imagination and your pocketbook." The benefits of automation may indeed appear so attractive that I&R agencies may overlook the negative aspects of automation, including higher financial costs than anticipated, a problem of lost access points regardless of how well the new automated system may function, and political costs that may occur if the staff proves incapable of converting the data to a machine-readable format. Hardware considerations that entail computers, microprocessors, hard disks, monitors, and graphics all represent major investments. Serious consideration must always be given to adequate provision for "backup" of data, which is a major factor in all automated operations. The advice given by Manikowski for database management is "to train your staff to back up your data every day that the database is edited, allow them sufficient time to do it, and then police them ruthlessly." A more detailed discussion on database management is presented in chapter 7.

According to Laura Zimmerman (in chap. 7), "training users of I&R data systems should include manuals that explain how the software works, in addition to 'hands-on training,' which tends to be the fastest way to get new users up to speed." Ideally, when a worker returns from training an immediate opportunity should be made available to use the live system or a practice system. In addition to developing, instituting, and operating computerized I&R systems is the need to modify operating systems as time and experience may indicate.

TRAINING PROGRAMS

Experience has indicated the advisability of offering training programs to administrators prior to staff training to familiarize them with the content of the program and to elicit their reactions and suggestions. The interest of top-level administrators is vital, particularly when staff members may become reluctant and even resistant to participating in predesigned I&R training programs. Another helpful suggestion is that staff participation in the initial planning of the training program can significantly reduce the resistance encountered when staff are confronted with a packaged training program. Inclusion of staff in the planning and implementation of training programs can considerably mitigate against the not uncommon problem of burnout, which may occur when staff is not sufficiently prepared to respond to heavy service demands, particularly in situations which involve crisis conditions.

Some beginnings have been made to provide academic instruction in I&R programs in a selected number of colleges and universities. Varying educational and training programs designed to prepare professionals for I&R program development and service provision were introduced in a limited number of graduate programs in the early 1970s. At the Adelphi University School of Social Work, I&R field internships and research projects in community development were designed for graduate and undergraduate students as early as 1971. In the mid-1970s, the Graduate School of Library Science at the University of Toledo offered a Community Information Specialist Program for library students interested in I&R community services. At Columbia University, faculty members from the library school provided instruction on I&R to both social work and library students under a federally funded program.

As I&R programs have continued to expand with the profound impact of information technology in gaining access to services, requirements for technical expertise in I&R operations have increased concurrently with other professional skills including organizational management, supervision, consultation, program development, and interorganizational expertise. The premise is that human helping skills are paramount and that information technology is capable of advancing "the human touch." The publication of I&R standards and criteria for professional performance have contributed to a clearer understanding of the professional conduct required for I&R quality service. A significant benefit of accreditation is the requirement for a professional review by qualified experts who examine and monitor I&R programs to assure the maintenance of standards for quality services (AIRS, 2000).

Though training programs for I&R services differ according to the individual agency settings, goals, and resources, fundamentals of I&R training tend to pertain to all I&R operations irrespective of settings and regional differences. Even for highly experienced staff, ongoing training courses in I&R expertise are essential to refine service delivery skills and maintain updated information on changes in policies, procedures, and relevant legislation. Developing working relationships with legislators in regard to community are mutually beneficial. Training in outreach and public relations programs is vital to publicize I&R programs and to reach potential clientele.

Because of the new and unprecedented capabilities of information technology to promote the organization and delivery of human services, I&R providers are not only expected, but required, to become familiar with the application of technology in I&R operations. In fact, without knowledge of the current and potential capabilities of information systems, communication techniques, and computer technology efforts to improve access through I&R may not operate with maximum effectiveness. New demands for managers with technological expertise and professional experience in the human services are increasingly sought, and will continue to be in demand. To meet changing needs and shifting service priorities, I&R training programs have developed a variety of on-the-job or in-service training programs. Irrespective of the setting of the I&R service, all staff require ongoing training in I&R expertise. Training programs also involve support staff, including secretaries, who answer the telephones, and maintenance staff, who may find it necessary to respond to an urgent phone call or an emergency drop-in after agency hours.

INSTRUCTIONAL MATERIALS

Since the early 1970s, a growing literature on I&R has begun to emerge to meet the informational and instructional needs of I&R training. During the early 1970s, Nicholas Long made a significant contribution to I&R training by editing a series of working drafts and prescriptive manuals on conducting I&R operations. (Interstudy, 1974). By 1979, various manuals and handbooks that dealt with direct client services and agency-specific procedures were used in educational and training programs. In response to the rapidly growing I&R programs in public libraries, Jones (1978) published a guide for librarians based on her I&R experience with the The Information Place (TIP) program at the Detroit Public Library. Focused primarily on training volunteers and paraprofessionals in a hypothetical, medium-sized urban community, Mathews and Fawcett (1981) offered some guidelines for staff training and program development. A highly popular 1969 movie, which dealt with various aspects of I&R service delivery, was *Tell Me Where to Turn*, produced by U.S. Public Affairs Committee in 1973. In 1979 a programmed self-help training course on I&R was published by United Way in the form of a workbook with an accompanying set of cassettes to guide the beginner in I&R operations.

A vital aspect of the professionalism of I&R services is the range of publications produced by AIRS. Since its first journal in 1979, AIRS has established itself as a professional agency with the continued publication of its journal and by issuing updated newsletters. In 1992 Norman Maas and Dick Manikowski of the Detroit Public Library coedited a comprehensive computerized bibliography that was also published in the AIRS journal (Maas & Manikowski, 1992). Continuous updates of this bibliography are compiled by Manikowski and intermittently published in the AIRS journal. The published bibliographies represent an essential professional contribution to the literature that deals with a wide range of subjects relevant to I&R.

Instructional materials that pertain to the AIRS/INFO LINE Taxonomy of Human Services include a comprehensive human services indexing system that was developed by Georgia Sales. A completely revised publication of *STANDARDS for Professional Information and Referral* (AIRS, 2000) reflects the growth and sophistication of information and referral services since the prior edition in 1981. A two-volume set of comprehensive training manuals is known as the ABCs of I&R. The first volume

includes individual study guides and instructions on basic I&R competencies, working with special populations, the role of I&R in times of disaster, and other practice areas. The second volume provides instructions
for trainers using templates and overhead projections. A general information source on the organizational mission and a discussion of the main
functions of an I&R agency are included in a 1995 booklet published by
AIRS and titled *Out of the Shadows*. Individual I&R agencies have also
published their own agency manuals, some of which are available for purchase. The expansion of the literature and instructional materials is a vital
feature of the new professionalism of I&R.

CONCLUSIONS

The quality of an I&R program hinges on the ability of its trained staff to
operate a reliable and responsible I&R service in accordance with the professional standards that have been formulated for I&R service provision.
To meet the learning needs of the different levels of staff, including volunteers, paraprofessional, and professionals an ongoing training program
is essential to guide the I&R agency in the initiation and operation of I&R
services. Opportunity to learn and apply relevant aspects of Information
Technology are of singular importance in the current practice of I&R.
Chapter 9 discusses the accomplishments of I&R as viewed retrospec-
tively, with a consideration of caveats and constraints that I&R programs
present. A giant leap into future developments of new routes to human
services is discussed prospectively.

REFERENCES

AIRS. (1996). *CIRS Application Packet*. Seattle, WA: AIRS.
AIRS. (2000). STANDARDS For Professional Information and Referral. Seattle,
    WA: AIRS.
AIRS Newsletter (September/October, 1984). Detroit resident vote to keep the doors
    open; assure future of local library system, TIP service. Vol. XII, No. 5, (1).
Childers, T. (1984). *Information and referral: Public libraries*. Norwood, NJ: Ablex
    Publishing Corporation.
Cueny, D., & Sales, G. (2000). AIRS launches new certification program for resource
    specialists. *AIRS Newsletter, 24*, 2, 6.
Drucker, P. F. (1995). *Managing in a time of great change*. New York: Truman Talley
    Books/Dutton.
Frederico, R. C. (1990). *Social welfare in today's world*. New York: McGraw Hill
    Publishing Co.

Gaines, E. (1980). Let's return to traditional library service· Facing the failure of social experimentation. *Wilson Library Bulletin, 55,* 50–53.

Gilbert, N., & Specht, H. (1974). *Dimensions of social welfare policy.* Englewood Cliffs, NJ: Prentice Hall.

Goldenberg, A. C. (1986). *1986 AIRS survey-professional training and education. Graduate level training programs in I&R.* Unpublished manuscript.

Hezel, L., & Jacobson, A. R. (1987). The nurse as a resource broker: A curriculum model. *Information and Referral: The Journal of the Alliance of Information and Referral Systems, 8* (1), 14–24.

Interstudy. (1974). *Information and referral services: Interviewing and information giving.* Minneapolis: Institute for Interdisciplinary studies of the American Rehabilitation Foundation. (ERIC Document Reproduction Service No. ED 055 635)

Jones, C. S. (Ed.). (1978). *Public library information and referral services.* Syracuse, NY: Gaylord.

Kahn, A. J., Kahn, A. J., Grossman, L., Bandler, J., Clark, F. R., Galkin, E., & Greenwalt, K. (1966). *Neighborhood information centers: A study and some proposals.* New York: Columbia University School of Social Work.

Kopecky, F. J. (1972). Office of Economic Opportunity community centers—a critical analysis. In C. A. Kronus, & L. Crowe (Eds.), *Libraries and information centers* (pp. 61–72). Urbana, IL: University of Illinois Press.

Levinson, R. W. (1996). Expanding I&R services for older adults in public libraries: Senior connections (1984–1985). *Information and Referral: The Journal of the Alliance of Information and Referral Systems, 18,* 21–40.

Long, N., Anderson, J., Burd, R., Mathis, M. E., & Todd, S. P., (1974). *Information and Referral Centers: A functional analysis,* (3rd ed.). (DHEW Publication No. OHD 75-20235). Minneapolis, MN: Interstudy.

Maas, N., & Manikowski, D. (Eds.). (1992). *Comprehensive bibliography of the literature of Information and Referral.* Information and Referral: The Journal of the Alliance of Information and Referral Systems, 14, Author.

Manikowski, D. (1990). Choosing an automated referral system. *Information and Referral: The Journal of the Alliance of Information and Referral Systems, 12* (1–2), 1–15.

Mathews, M. R., & Fawcett, S. B. (1981). *Matching clients and services: Information and referral.* Beverly Hills, CA: Sage.

National Commission on Library and Information Science. (1983). *Final Report of the Community Information and Referral Task Force.* Washington, DC: Community Information and Referral Services.

PART IV

Epilogue

CHAPTER 9

Viewing I&R in a New Millennium

Despite its relatively short history as a public policy,
I&R has achieved a central role in the social services.
The rate of diffusion and adoption of I&R activities
has been more rapid than for most innovations.
Shanahan, Gargan, & Apple, 1983

Although the roots of I&R can be traced to the early social service organizations of the 18th century, I&R, as an organizational entity, represents a brief history of slightly more than four decades. This relatively new phenomenon in the complex field of human services has been challenged by experts regarding future directions. In the first issue of the AIRS journal in 1979, Nick Long (1979) of Interstudy Associates raised these cogent questions regarding "Information and Referral Services in the 1980s: Where should they go? Who should lead? Will anyone follow?" Fourteen years later, Peter Aberg and Gil Evans (1993) asked the following question at the Annual 1992 AIRS Conference; "Whither I&R?" Many of the forecasts that were presented then have been realized, other predictions remain to be seen. With the advent of the new millennium, this concluding chapter takes a retrospective view on the attainments of I&R within a history of less than a half century, and looks ahead prospectively to a new millennium, while acknowledging some of the caveats and constraints that merit consideration.

A RETROSPECTIVE VIEW

I&R has evolved from an interested group of dedicated volunteers in the early 1960s to a growing corps of service providers who represent all levels of staff. The development and expansion of I&R over the past four

163

decades are a credit to the vision and commitment of the early founders of the I&R movement. Representing various communities throughout the United States, these volunteers recognized the urgent need to facilitate access to human services within the complex systems of health and social services, collectively regarded as the human services.

Within the past two scores of years, I&R has expanded exponentially as a national and international social service with a level of sophistication and professionalism that combines universal access to human services and information technology, thereby opening up new routes to human services. Entering the new millennium, I&R services now operate on all levels including local, state, regional, provincial, national, and international levels.

THE NATIONAL I&R TRIAD

The growth and expansion of I&R services clearly reflect the leadership of The National I&R TRIAD—namely the United Way of America (UWA), the Administration on Aging (AoA), and the Alliance of Information and Referral Systems (AIRS). Since the early 1960s each of these organizations has been concurrently involved in the promotion and expansion of I&R services within their own organizations as well as in "creative partnerships" with one another. Thanks to the cooperation and collaboration of these three nationwide organizations since the decade of the 1960s, dramatic progress has been made in the advancement of I&R as a vital professional service.

THE IMPACT OF AUTOMATION

A major factor in the dramatic growth of I&R services, particularly since the mid-1980s, has been the enormous gains in computerization and the explosive development of information technology, which has advanced the field of I&R in new and unprecedented ways. Shared databases have promoted a level of interorganizational cooperation and collaboration, which have contributed to new and sophisticated information systems. Advancements in the application of hardware and software have promoted new database systems and opportunities for data sharing in unprecedented ways. Negroponte (1995) forecasts that because of "the empowering nature of 'being digital,' the access, the mobility, and the ability to affect change re what will make the future so different from the present."

TAXONOMY: A COMMON LANGUAGE

The development of a universal taxonomy in the field of I&R has created new opportunities to utilize a common language for the universal identification and classification of health and social services. The availability of the taxonomy ensures a common language for the identification of services, with definitions that follow a hierarchical classification of terms. The flexibility and the ease in utilizing the taxonomy provide an opportunity for "indexing terms" with a facility that has not existed heretofore in the social services, thus creating new opportunities for universal service identification and a common basis for social research.

ATTAINMENT OF PROFESSIONALISM

Attainments of professionalism in the decade of the 1990s represent a significant accomplishment in the field of I&R. A newly defined and updated set of formally approved standards for professional I&R practice specifies the dimensions, the latitude, and the boundaries of I&R professionals. By meeting required qualifications for professional practice, I&R providers can now attain professional certification with the designation of Certified Information Referral Specialist (CIRS). Professionalism in I&R has been further advanced in accordance with regulations delineated by AIRs for agency accreditation.

RESPONSES TO CRISIS AND DISASTER

Given the increased availability of shared databases and service networks to respond to emergency conditions, I&R services have demonstrated the capability to respond with immediacy and planfulness to emergencies, disasters, and catastrophes. Under disaster conditions, I&R agencies have demonstrated the effectiveness of entering into helping partnerships with other organizations. Providers of I&R services have also exercised expertise to apply professional helping skills in disaster *planning* as well as in disaster *aid*, thereby defining a new role for I&R under emergency conditions.

THE 211 UNIVERSAL TELEPHONE SERVICE

An enormous achievement in I&R developments has been the approval of the national 211 universal telephone services. Thanks to the political wisdom of I&R advocates in gaining this approval from the U.S. Federal

Communication Committee, the field of I&R has achieved the opportunity to provide universal access services to all callers. The establishment of the 211 number has heralded a new era in the history of I&R developments. The success in attaining this access system also presents a challenge to individual communities in instituting this phone service in local communities. This will require that individual communities will need to adapt 211 in accordance with their specific locales.

INTERNATIONAL I&R DEVELOPMENTS

The British system of Citizens Advice Bureaus, which predates the American I&R movement by at least 20 years, demonstrated the universality of need for organized access systems for "information, advice, and counsel." According to Levinson and Haynes (1984), a select number of other countries have patterned their access systems similar to the CAB model. A recent development in international I&R extends I&R services in North America. Under the presidency of Gil Evans (2000a, 2000b), a former president of AIRS, the newly organized Inform Canada Federation programs have now been extended to include the continent of North America.

A vital aspect of international I&R is the growing membership of the American military in AIRS. With representation from all branches of the armed forces, military personnel are involved in carrying out I&R programs utilizing both military and civilian personnel. Attendance of the military at annual AIRS conferences has increased significantly since the mid-1980s as has the participation of I&R personnel in family support centers. Military personnel share a common goal with all other I&R operators in their commitment to quality as CIRS providers. The availability of I&R services is of central importance to the person and to the family in the military, particularly when family readiness is primary for deployment.

CAVEATS AND CONSTRAINTS

Despite the extraordinary capabilities and wonders of cyberspace, the computer still remains "a tool." In his formal address at the seventh national conference of AIRS, Ward, a guest speaker from England, reminded the AIRS assemblage that "the computer is only a tool that cannot see a disability, a smile, or a tear" (AIRS, 1985). Other authorities have also expressed concern that there is an inherent danger that we may forsake our social values and cultural aspirations and become a "technopoly" (Postman, 1992). Other warnings have been sounded by Shenk (1995), who expresses concern that we may be the victims of *information overload* and therefore become subject to "data smog." Another problem that threatens our new information era is that knowledge can be easily turned into property with the inherent danger that freely shared knowledge may become the property of private business interests (Shulman, 1999). As noted by Sales (2000), we need to be alert for the threat of the proprietary organization, which sees a way to make a profit on community information, often using the very data we maintain.

According to Kranich (2001), president of the American Library Association, a serious social concern is the so-called digital divide, whereby many low-income, minority, disabled, rural, and inner-city groups are falling behind in their ownership of computers and their access to telecommunications networks. Differential access to computer capabilities and lack of necessary skills are also serious barriers to acquiring available information. Even for those who have the computer skills, one needs to be aware that not all advice on health care and suggested medications, remedies, and therapies are necessarily valid or reliable. One needs to exercise careful judgment and discernment. As for the physical concerns in computer utilization, Manikowski (2000) offers advice on how to counteract the hazards and risks inherent in the operation of computers. Faulty vision, the use of improper lighting, negligent posture, improper hand operations on the keyboard, and prolonged sessions may all contribute to physical problems.

Even though data derived from computers can serve as a barometer to spot trends, identify needs and gaps, and reflect changing priorities, one cannot presume that I&R has the capacity to overcome serious service gaps and inadequacies that exist in social service systems. I&R does not actually solve social problems nor should I&R organizations be regarded as "cause agencies." As a social service modality, I&R services cannot actually solve the broad societal problems of poverty, unemployment, and discrimination. However, data derived from I&R services can indicate the magnitude and gravity of existing problems, and thereby provide a highly valuable barometer of social concerns.

A PROSPECTIVE VIEW

A CHANGING DEMOGRAPHY

The future of all social services, including I&R, will be affected by significant changes that are due to occur in the demography and the characteristics of the population. In the next 10 years the aging of the population, the movement of the baby boomers through the life cycle, and the increasing ethnic and cultural diversity of the population will profoundly alter demands for social services, including I&R services. The dramatic increase in the extension of longevity and the subsequent chronicity of the older population are vital factors in considering service provision for a changing population.

SELF-HELP/SELF-EMPOWERMENT

As automated information systems will continue to be used more extensively, computerized systems will become increasingly "user-friendly." Analogous to the book-borrowing patron of the public library, who independently selects books and other published materials, the information seeker possesses or can quite readily acquire the ability to retrieve data and extract information from data systems quite independently. Through home-based computerized equipment, including interactive videotext and cable, the I&R end user has unprecedented opportunities for self-help.

The Internet will continue to be a vital tool in the daily lives of increasing numbers of people. According to a recent federal report, cited in the AIRS journal, more than half of all Americans use the Internet (White & Madara, 2000). Telecommunications will continue to increase the opportunity for people to advocate for their own needs and interests, thereby providing a stronger sense of self-empowerment.

I&R: FOCUS ON COMMUNITY

As I&R programs continue to proliferate on all levels of operation, it is vital that the local community be considered of primary importance. The effectiveness of securing I&R within the local community has always been a major interest. The task ahead will be how to assure that local residents will have access to needed information within their local settings. Historically, both Nicholas Long (1973) and Georgia Sales (2000) have put prime emphasis on the accessibility of data in the local community. It is expected that kiosks will be more widely used as public information sources within local communities. I&R programs will increasingly be made available to serve people wherever they meet or congregate, such as shopping plazas, train stations, churches, city halls and recreation centers. Local community schools, hospitals, police and fire departments, and public libraries will also participate in what will be community-based I&R services. Moreover, I&R services will continue to gain prominence and expand at the workplace as more social welfare programs are located in industry for the mutual benefit of employees and company management. By utilizing computer modalities, such as e-mail, listservs, chat rooms, and the Internet, automation also has the capacity to create "virtual communities," whereby people share interests and commonalities, irrespective of geographic boundaries.

STAFFING & TRAINING

The availability of systematized access to human services will impact on all health and social services to the extent that providers will have the need to become more knowledgeable and skilled to seek out available and appropriate resources. Staff training for agencies and academic orientations for professional service providers will become far more available to gain the knowledge and skills required for professional practice. Programs of distance education and teleconferencing will promote the availability of educational opportunities at the learner's convenience regardless of time and place since participants can log on to courses any time, any place, worldwide.

NEW FUNDING PATTERNS

In the assurance of universal access to services, careful consideration must be given at all times to the inclusion-exclusion criteria, which determine choices of resources in the databases and a guarding of the social programs that serve the best interests of the public. However, a reality is that the field of I&R is also becoming more involved in the for-profit sector to the extent that the for-profit sector may offer increasing numbers of choices. I&R agencies have come to recognize that the for-profit sectors can offer choices that are not available in the voluntary nonprofit sectors. Funding resources will continue to represent a vast variety of financing sources including the government, charitable funds, corporate funds, agency fees for services, and revenues obtained from sales of agency directories.

FOCUS ON RESEARCH

Research in the field of I&R will be significantly enhanced with the availability of shared databases, which suggests areas for investigation, such as the incidence and gravity of specific social problems, client tracking, identification of target populations, and comparative strategies for effective service delivery. The utilization of an indexed taxonomy also provides research opportunities to study selected services according to defined parameters of service agendas. The sanction to establish the 211 telephone system presents a challenging research opportunity for any given community. Research on model I&R systems are projected to spot trends, identify needs and gaps, and reflect changing priorities. The extent to which I&R may be able to reconceptualize or in any way reshape the social welfare system will clearly depend upon the extent of political endorsement and fiscal support that can be mustered.

IMPACT ON HUMAN SERVICES

The continued expansion of I&R services on all levels will effect greater communication between I&R services and the existing social service infrastructure. Rather than inventing new resources, service organizations will rely on I&R services, as indicated. Interagency networking will provide increased opportunity to deliver more comprehensive services, thereby benefiting the client as well as the social agency. The expanded professionalism that the field of I&R has attained will also command greater recognition on behalf of service providers in other helping professions. Given the availability and accessibility of I&R services, agencies will be interested in using the available services rather than inventing other service organizations.

A GLOBAL INFORMATION SOCIETY

Thanks to the wonders of automation and the new modes of communication, more instantaneously shared information throughout planet earth and outer space has become available. The extent to which I&R can or will function as an organized international service remains to be developed. It has been acknowledged that in a world of mobile population groups, cross-national information and referral services can be appropriately used to assist displaced citizens, refugee groups, and newly arrived minorities with access to needed resources. International health issues and crisis conditions due to natural disasters and social catastrophes can be significantly ameliorated given the availability and accessibility to reach and utilize organized systems of health and social services. As to the potentialities of future developments in I&R, Georgia Sales (2000) observed that "the opportunities for expanding the role of information and referral may be limited only by the boundaries of our creativity."

REFERENCES

Aberg, P., & Evans, G. (1993). *Whither I&R?* Orlando, FL: AIRS 1992 Conference Workshop.

AIRS Newsletter. (1985). Englishman addresses 7th national conference on issues advices and information services will face. *AIRS Newsletter: Alliance of Information and Referral Systems, XII* (3), 1.

Evans, G. (2000a). Report from the Great white North. *AIRS Newsletter: Alliance of Information and Referral Systems, XXIV* (2), 18.

Evans, G. (2000b). Report from the Great white North. *AIRS Newsletter: Alliance of Information and Referral Systems, XXIV* (4), 17.

Kranich, N. (January 2001). Ensuring information equity in the digital age. *American Libraries, 32* (1), 7.

Levinson, R. W., & Haynes, K. S. (1984). *Accessing human services: International perspectives.* Beverly Hills: Sage.

Long, N. (1973). Information and Referral Services. A short history and some recommendations. *The Social Service Review, 47* (1), 49–62.

Long, N. (1979). Information and referral services in the 1980s: Where should they go? Who should lead? Will anyone follow? *Information and Referral: The Journal of the Alliance of Information and Referral Services, 1* (1), 1–24.

Manikowski, D. (2000). Setting inclusion/exclusion criteria: Determining the scope of a resource file. *Information and Referral: The Journal of the Alliance of Information and Referral Systems, 22* (9), 111–138.

Negroponte, N. (1995). *Being digital.* New York: Vintage Books.

Postman, N. (1992). *Technopoly: The surrender of culture to technology.* New York: Knopf.

Sales, G. (2000). I&R leadership in the information age. *Information and Referral: The Journal of the Alliance of Information and Referral Systems, 22,* 139–158.

Shanahan, J. L., Gargan, J. J., & Apple, N. (1983). *Building model I&R systems: A bridge to the future.* Akron, OH: Alliance of Information and Referral Systems, Inc.

Shenk, D. (1997). *Data smog.* New York: HarperCollins.

Shulman, S. (1999). *Owning the future*. New York: Houghton Mifflin.

White, J. W., & Madara, E. (2000). Online mutual support groups: Identifying and tapping new I&R resources. *Self-help clearing houses*. Cedar Krolls: NJ. *Information and Referral: The Journal of the Alliance of Information and Referral Systems, 22,* 63–82.

I&R: A Chronology (1860–2000)

1860s	Charity Organization Societies—I&R-type services for individuals and families
1870's	Settlement Houses—I&R-type services for neighborhood communities
1912	United Way Chapter in Cleveland—Community Directory Service (I&R function)
1914	American Red Cross Emergency Services—I&R-type training program
1939	Citizens Advice Bureaus established during World War II in England, Scotland, and North Wales
1946	U.S. Veterans Information Centers (VICS)
1948	Veterans Bureau established
1962	National Easter Seal—I&R Community programs for the disabled
1964	Social Action Programs—community-based I&R services focused on "the right to know"
1965	Creation of the Office of the Administration on Aging (AoA) under the Older American Act (OAA) of 1965
1967	Bloksberg & Caso study—first comprehensive national survey of I&R
1969	First I&R library-based I&R program in Enoch Pratt Library in Maryland
1971	I&R model program in Detroit, Michigan, known as TIP (The Information Place)
1971	United Way published the first National Standards for I&R
1972–1978	I&R roundtables sponsored by United Way at the annual National Conferences on Social Welfare

1972	United Way published the first national service classification system known as UWASIS—the United Way of America Service Identification System. Reformulation of this system in 1976 known as UWASIS II
1973	AIRS established as an independent incorporated organization
1974	AoA set minimum requirements and guidelines for I&R services
1974	AIRS first publication of National Standards
1975	Title XX of the Social Security Act—provided I&R training programs to states
1977	First published issue of AIRS newsletter
1978	Book by Clara Jones—A prescriptive overview of library-based I&R operations
1979	AIRS first national conference in Phoenix, Arizona
1972–1979	Corazon Estava Doyle—First national volunteer executive director of AIRS
1979	Publication of the first issue of the AIRS journal
1983	Special issue of AIRS journal on computerization in I&R services
1983	Model study of Information and Referral Systems—A Bridge to the Future
1985	AoA grant to Adelphi University School of Social Work to conduct Senior Connections—a library-based I&R program for older volunteers, students, librarians, and social workers
1987	First publication of INFO LINE Taxonomy of Human Services—Georgia Sales, Director
1988	Textbook on Information and Referral Networks: *Doorways to Human Services*. Springer. First edition. Risha W. Levinson, author
1989	Development of the Certified Information and Referral Specialist model (CIRS)
1990	A self-study manual for I&R Services—an AIRS publication
1991	Eldercare Locator—national telephone service targeted to the aging—established by the Administration on Aging

1992	Comprehensive bibliography on I&R—coeditors: Norman L. Maas and Dick Manikowski. Published in the *Journal of the Alliance of Information and Referral Systems* (1992), Volume 14
1992	AoA cosponsorship with AIRS at Annual AIRS Conferences
1992	First attendance of the military at AIRS annual conference
1993	ABC's of I&R—10 Manuals—Edited by Ann Jacobson, LCSW
1994	A Taxonomy of Human Services: A conceptual framework with standardized terminology and definitions for the field
1995	*Out of the Shadows—Overview of I&R and AIRS*—An information guide
1996	AIRS received grant for membership to NERIN—National Emergency Response Information Network
1997	American Library Association, Public Library Associations—*Guidelines for Establishing Community Information and Referral Services in Public Libraries*. Edited by Norman L. Maas and Dick Manikowski
1998	25th Anniversary of AIRS (1973–1998)—Gil Evans, Warren Nance, and Hezel Smith
1998	The ABC's of I&R Volume I (A self-study guide). Volume II (A trainer's guide)
1999	Development of interorganizational networks in response to disaster aid services (INFORM, NERIN)
1999	AIRS Electronic Directory of Information and Referral Providers
1999	Creating a 211 Service: A Comprehensive Guide to Developing a 211 Information and Referral Service
2000 (April)	AIRS accreditation formally launched with I&R agencies
2000 (May)	Publication of Standards for Professional Information & Referral—4th edition
2000 (June)	Inform Canada Federation incorporated as a regional member of AIRS. Gil Evans, president
2000 (July 21)	U.S. Federal Communications Commission (FCC) approval of the national telephone dialing code—211

APPENDIX B-1

United Way of America (UWA): Changes in Total Numbers of I&R Agencies

Comparative Data: 1984 and 2000

UWA	1985	2000	Change (%)
1 Alabama	7	10	43
2 Alaska	0	1	
3 Arizona	3	2	–33
4 Arkansas	2	9	350
5 California	15	26	73
6 Colorado	8	11	38
7 Connecticut	13	1	-92
8 Delaware	1	1	0
9 District of Columbia	0	—	—
10 Florida	16	27	69
11 Georgia	7	11	57
12 Hawaii	2	4	100
13 Idaho	3	7	133
14 Illinois	14	18	29
15 Indiana	13	18	38
16 Iowa	9	10	11
17 Kansas	6	7	17
18 Kentucky	4	6	50

19	Louisiana	4	7	75
20	Maine	1	4	300
21	Maryland	3	1	-67
22	Massachusetts	7	17	143
23	Michigan	14	19	36
24	Minnesota	8	12	50
25	Mississippi	7	9	29
26	Missouri	7	6	-14
27	Montana	3	5	67
28	Nebraska	2	6	200
29	Nevada	2	2	0
30	New Hampshire	7	8	14
31	New Jersey	17	23	35
32	New Mexico	2	4	100
33	New York	16	20	25
34	North Carolina	10	25	150
35	North Dakota	1	4	300
36	Ohio	31	28	-10
37	Oklahoma	6	9	50
38	Oregon	5	7	40
39	Pennsylvania	22	23	5
40	Rhode Island	1	1	0
41	South Carolina	4	10	150
42	South Dakota	2	2	0
43	Tennessee	3	11	267
44	Texas	24	32	33
45	Utah	2	3	50
46	Vermont	0	1	
47	Virginia	8	14	75
48	Washington	11	13	18
49	West Virginia	4	7	75
50	Wisconsin	11	16	45
51	Wyoming	1	4	300
	Total:	**369**	**522**	**41**

Sources: United Way 1985 Directory of Information and Referral Services.
         Alexandria, VA: United Way of America
         Where to call for Help - A nationwide Directory for United Way I&R Services—2001.

APPENDIX B-2

Administration on Aging (AoA): Changes in Total Numbers of I&R Agencies

Comparative Data: 1985 and 1999

	AoA	1985	1999	Change (%)
1	Alabama	13	12	−8
2	Alaska	1	1	0
3	Arizona	8	8	0
4	Arkansas	8	8	0
5	California	33	33	0
6	Colorado	15	14	−7
7	Connecticut	5	5	0
8	Delaware	1	1	0
9	District of Columbia	1	1	0
10	Florida	11	11	0
11	Georgia	18	18	0
12	Hawaii	4	4	0
13	Idaho	6	6	0
14	Illinois	13	13	0
15	Indiana	16	15	−6
16	Iowa	13	16	23
17	Kansas	11	11	0
18	Kentucky	15	15	0

19	Louisiana	42	36	−14
20	Maine	5	5	0
21	Maryland	18	19	6
22	Massachusetts	23	23	0
23	Michigan	14	14	0
24	Minnesota	14	12	−14
25	Mississippi	10	10	0
26	Missouri	10	10	0
27	Montana	11	11	0
28	Nebraska	8	8	0
29	Nevada	1	1	0
30	New Hampshire	1	1	0
31	New Jersey	21	21	0
32	New Mexico	4	6	50
33	New York	61	59	−3
34	North Carolina	18	18	0
35	North Dakota	1	1	0
36	Ohio	12	11	−8
37	Oklahoma	11	11	0
38	Oregon	18	18	0
39	Pennsylvania	50	52	4
40	Rhode Island	1	1	0
41	South Carolina	15	10	−33
42	South Dakota	1	1	0
43	Tennessee	9	9	0
44	Texas	28	28	0
45	Utah	13	12	−8
46	Vermont	5	5	0
47	Virginia	26	25	−4
48	Washington	13	13	0
49	West Virginia	11	4	−64
50	Wisconsin	6	6	0
51	Wyoming	1	1	0
	Total:	**674**	**654**	**−3**

Sources: *A Directory of State and Area Agencies on Aging,* 4th ed. (1985 March).
State Committee on Aging, House of Representatives, Ninety-ninth Congress.
Washington, DC: U.S. Government Printing Office. (Pub. No. 99-490.)
National Directory for Eldercare I&R, 2000–2001.

APPENDIX B-3

Alliance of Information and Referral Systems, Inc. (AIRS): Changes in Total Numbers of Agencies

Comparative Data: 1984 & 1996

AIRS		1984	1995–96	Change (%)
1	Alabama	2	35	1650
2	Alaska	1	1	0
3	Arizona	3	32	967
4	Arkansas	7	33	371
5	California	52	181	248
6	Colorado	9	39	333
7	Connecticut	8	26	225
8	Delaware	2	6	200
9	District of Columbia	2	—	—
10	Florida	17	121	612
11	Georgia	6	45	650
12	Hawaii	4	26	550
13	Idaho	6	33	450
14	Illinois	31	115	271
15	Indiana	20	77	285
16	Iowa	11	28	155
17	Kansas	15	31	107
18	Kentucky	4	12	200
19	Louisiana	12	20	67

20	Maine	2	21	950
21	Maryland	20	48	140
22	Massachusetts	15	59	293
23	Michigan	18	90	400
24	Minnesota	9	45	400
25	Mississippi	7	16	129
26	Missouri	13	26	100
27	Montana	3	26	767
28	Nebraska	8	20	150
29	Nevada	1	10	900
30	New Hampshire	7	7	0
31	New Jersey	25	76	204
32	New Mexico	3	25	733
33	New York	45	90	100
34	North Carolina	11	65	491
35	North Dakota	4	7	75
36	Ohio	43	124	188
37	Oklahoma	7	32	357
38	Oregon	12	158	1217
39	Pennsylvania	32	105	228
40	Rhode Island	2	11	450
41	South Carolina	2	16	700
42	South Dakota	4	9	125
43	Tennessee	3	8	167
44	Texas	32	111	247
45	Utah	10	14	40
46	Vermont	2	16	700
47	Virginia	12	47	292
48	Washington	12	56	367
49	West Virginia	4	15	275
50	Wisconsin	10	46	360
51	Wyoming	4	3	−25
	Total:	**594**	**2263**	**281**

Sources: —Alliance of Information & Referral Services Inc. (1984).
   Directory of information and referral services in the United States and Canada. Indianapolis: Author.
   —Directory of AIRS & United Way of America 1995–96 Joliet, IL.

APPENDIX C

Comparative State Totals of I&R Agencies Reported by AIRS According to Regional Areas (1984–1996)

Northwest	Total Agencies	
	1984–1985	1995–1996
Alaska	1	1
Idaho	6	33
Montana	3	26
Oregon	12	158
Washington	12	56
Wyoming	4	3
Region Total	**38**	**277**
Nationwide Comparison	**6%**	**12%**

North Central	Total Agencies	
	1984–1985	**1995–1996**
Illinois	31	115
Iowa	11	28
Kansas	15	31
Minnesota	9	45
Missouri	13	26
Nebraska	8	20
North Dakota	4	7
South Dakota	4	9
Wisconsin	10	46
Region Total	**105**	**327**
Nationwide Comparison	**18%**	**14%**

Southwest	Total Agencies	
	1984–1985	**1995–1996**
Arizona	3	32
California	52	181
Colorado	9	39
Hawaii	4	26
Nevada	1	10
New Mexico	3	25
Utah	10	14
Region Total	**82**	**327**
Nationwide Comparison	**14%**	**14%**

South Central	Total Agencies	
	1984–1985	1995–1996
Arkansas	7	33
Louisiana	12	20
Oklahoma	7	32
Texas	32	111
Region Total	**58**	**196**
Nationwide Comparison	**10%**	**9%**

Nationwide Data	1984–1985	1995–1996
As reported by AIRS	7	33

Northeast	Total Agencies	
	1984–1985	1995–1996
Connecticut	8	26
Delaware	2	6
District of Columbia	2	–
Indiana	20	77
Maine	2	21
Maryland	20	48
Massachusetts	15	59
Michigan	18	90
New Hampshire	7	7
New Jersey	25	76
New York	45	90
Ohio	43	124
Pennsylvania	32	105
Rhode Island	2	11
Vermont	2	16
Region Total	**243**	**756**
Nationwide Comparison	**41%**	**33%**

Southeast	Total Agencies	
	1984–1985	**1995–1996**
Alabama	2	35
Florida	17	121
Georgia	6	45
Kentucky	4	12
Mississippi	7	16
North Carolina	11	65
South Carolina	2	16
Tennessee	3	8
Virginia	12	47
West Virginia	4	15
Region Total	**68**	**380**
Nationwide Comparison	**11%**	**17%**

APPENDIX D

Suggested Web Sites

Compiled by Laura I. Zimmerman, PhD

Alliance for Information and Referral Services of New Jersey
http://www.aclink.org/AIRS-NJ/
Atlanta, Georgia
http://www.unitedwayatl.org/findhelp/index.htm
British Columbia Alliance for Information and Referral Services
http://www.vcn.bc.ca/bcairs/
California Alliance for Information and Referral Services
http://www.infoline-la.org/cairs/CAIRS/CAIRS.htm
City of Calgary, Alberta—http://www.gov.calgary.ab.ca/81/info/index.html
Community Information and Referral, Central and North Arizona—
http://www.cirs.org/
First White Plains, New York—http://www.firstwp.org/
Florida Alliance for Information and Referral Services
http://www.flairs.org/
Information and Referral Network Indianapolis, Indiana
http://www.irni.org/
Information and Referral Resource Network—http://www.ir-net.com/
index.html
Information & Referral, Vancouver, Washington—http://www.irccv.
org/i&r/idx_i&r.htm
Iowa AIRS—http://www.iowaairs.org/
Maryland Information and Referral Providers Council
http://www.angelfire.com/md2/mirpc/

Mid-East Commission, Washington, NC—http://www.mecaaa.org/
Midwest Information and Referral Service Alliance
    http://www.deltaboogie.com/mirsa/
Minnesota Information and Referral Alliance
    http://www.firstcall-mn.org/MIRA/index.html
National Alliance for Information and Referral Systems
    http://www.airs.org/
National Association for Child Care Resource and Referral
    http://www.naccrra.net/
New York Alliance for Information and Referral Systems
    http://www.nysairs.org/
North Carolina Alliance for Information and Referral Services
    http://www.angelfire.com/nc/ncairs/
Northern California Council for the Community
    http://www.ncccsf.org/i_and_r/index.html
Northwest Alliance for Information and Referral Systems
    http://www.nwairs.org/
Texas Information and Referral Network
    http://www.hhsc.state.tx.us/tirn/tirnhome.htm
United Way of Southern Nevada
    http://uwaysn.communityos.org/

Appendix E

Summary of I&R Standards*

I. SERVICE DELIVERY

The standards in Section I describe the service delivery functions essential for providing information and referral and assuring access for all, including a brief individual assessment of need; a blend of information, referral and advocacy in order to link the person to the appropriate service; and follow-up, as required.

STANDARD 1: INFORMATION PROVISION

The I&R service shall provide information to an inquirer in response to a direct request for such information. Information can range from a limited response (such as an organization's name, telephone number, and address) to detailed data about community service systems (such as explaining how a group intake system works for a particular agency), agency policies, and procedures for application.

STANDARD 2: REFERRAL PROVISION

The I&R service shall provide information and referral services in which the inquirer has one-to-one, human contact with an I&R specialist. The referral process consists of assessing the needs of the inquirer, identifying appropriate resources, assessing appropriate response modes, indicating organizations capable of meeting those needs, providing enough information about each organization to help inquirers make an informed choice, helping inquirers for whom services are unavailable by locating alterna-

---

* *STANDARDS For Professional Information and Referral*. Alliance of Information and Referral Systems (AIRS, 2000).

tive resources, and, when necessary, actively participating in linking the inquirer to needed services.

STANDARD 3: ADVOCACY/INTERVENTION

The I&R service shall offer advocacy to ensure that people receive the benefits and services to which they are entitled and that organizations within the established service delivery system meet the collective needs of the community. For purposes of these standards, "advocacy" does not include legislative advocacy (lobbying). All advocacy efforts shall be consistent with policies established by the governing body of the I&R service and shall proceed only with the permission of the inquirer.

STANDARD 4: FOLLOW-UP

The I&R service shall have a written policy which addresses the conditions under which follow-up must be conducted. The policy shall mandate follow-up with inquirers in endangerment situations and in situations where the specialist believes that the inquirer does not have the necessary capacity to follow through and resolve his or her problem and must specify a percentage of other inquiries for which follow-up is required. Additional assistance in locating or *using* services may be necessary.

II. RESOURCE DATABASE

The standards in Section 11 describe the requirement that the I&R service shall develop, maintain, and/or use an accurate, up-to-date resource database that contains an article about available community resources including detailed data on the services they provide and the conditions under which services are available. If the I&R service maintains a resource database, of Web Sites on the Internet, Resource Database Standards 5 through 9 still apply.

STANDARD 5: INCLUSION/EXCLUSION CRITERIA

The I&R service shall develop criteria for the inclusion or exclusion of agencies and programs in the resource database. These criteria shall be uniformly applied and published so that staff and the public will be aware of the scope and limitations of the database.

STANDARD 6: DATA ELEMENTS

A standardized profile shall be developed for each organization that is part of the local community service delivery system or other geographic area covered by the I&R service.

STANDARD 7: INDEXING THE RESOURCE DATABASE/SEARCH METHODS

Information in the resource database shall be indexed and accessible in ways that support the I&R process.

STANDARD 8: CLASSIFICATION SYSTEM (TAXONOMY)

The I&R service shall use a standard service classification system to facilitate retrieval of community resource information, to increase the reliability of planning data, to make evaluation processes consistent and reliable, and to facilitate national comparisons of data. Additional classification structures such as key words may supplement the taxonomy.

STANDARD 9: DATABASE MAINTENANCE

The resource database shall be updated through continuous revision or at intervals sufficiently frequent to ensure accuracy of information and comprehensiveness of its contents.

III. REPORTS AND MEASURES

The standards in Section III describe the inquirer data collection, analysis, and reporting functions of the I&R service.

STANDARD 10: INQUIRER DATA COLLECTION

The I&R service shall establish and use a system for collecting and organizing inquirer data that facilitates appropriate referrals and provides a basis for describing requests for service, identifying service gaps and overlaps, assisting with needs assessments, supporting the development of products, identifying issues for staff training, and facilitating the development of the resource information system. Inquirer data includes information gathered during follow-up as well as that acquired during the original contact.

STANDARD 11: DATA ANALYSIS AND REPORTING

The I&R service shall develop reports using inquirer data and/or data from the resource database to support community planning activities (or planning at other levels), internal analysis, and advocacy.

IV. COOPERATIVE RELATIONSHIPS

The standards in Section IV focus on the responsibilities of the I&R service to the local I&R system, the local community service delivery system, and state or provincial, regional, national, and international I&R networks.

STANDARD 12: COOPERATIVE RELATIONSHIPS WITHIN THE LOCAL I&R SYSTEM

In communities that have a multiplicity of comprehensive and specialized I&R providers, the I&R service shall develop cooperative working relationships to build a coordinated I&R system which ensures broad access to information and referral services, maximizes the utilization of existing I&R resources, avoids duplication of effort, and encourages seamless access to community resource information. I&R services within the system may choose to be "full service" programs performing all necessary I&R functions within their designated service area; or may prefer to partner with one or more I&R services to share those functions. (For example, one I&R service might build and maintain the resource database and another might assume responsibility for service delivery.)

STANDARD 13: COOPERATIVE RELATIONSHIPS WITHIN THE LOCAL SERVICE DELIVERY SYSTEM

The I&R service shall strive to develop cooperative working relationships with local service providers to build an integrated service delivery system that ensures broad access to community services, maximizes the utilization of existing resources, avoids duplication, of effort and gaps in services, and facilitates the ability of people who need services to easily find the most appropriate provider.

STANDARD 14: COOPERATIVE RELATIONSHIPS AMONG LOCAL, STATE OR PROVINCIAL, REGIONAL, NATIONAL AND INTERNATIONAL I&R PROVIDERS

Comprehensive and specialized I&R services at all geographic levels (local, state/provincial, regional, national, and international) shall strive to develop formal and informal working relationships with the objective of broadening the availability of information and referral to all inquirers, facilitating access to appropriate resources regardless of their origin and/or location, avoiding duplication of effort and funding, expanding the effectiveness of social analysis with more global information about needs and services, and augmenting the impact of advocacy efforts through coordination, where possible.

STANDARD 15: PARTICIPATION IN STATE OR PROVINCIAL, REGIONAL, NATIONAL, AND INTERNATIONAL I&R ASSOCIATIONS

The I&R service shall strive to strengthen state or provincial, regional, national, and international I&R networks by becoming active in planning, program development, advocacy, training, and other efforts at these levels.

V. ORGANIZATIONAL REQUIREMENTS

The standards in Section V describe the governance and administrative structure an I&R service needs to have in place in order for it to carry out its mission. Included are establishing itself as a legal entity, providing for ongoing program evaluation, developing policies and procedures that guide the organization, developing an organizational code of ethics, establishing sound fiscal practices, providing a conducive physical environment, managing personnel, providing for staff training, and increasing public awareness regarding the availability of information and referral services and their value to the community.

STANDARD 16: GOVERNANCE

The auspices under which the I&R service operates shall ensure the achievement of I&R goals and meet the stated goals of funders.

STANDARD 17: PERSONNEL ADMINISTRATION

The I&R service shall provide a framework and mechanisms for program and personnel management and administration that guarantee the continuity and consistency required for effective service delivery.

STANDARD 18: STAFF TRAINING

The I&R service shall have a training policy and make training available to paid and volunteer staff.

STANDARD 19: PROMOTION AND OUTREACH

The I&R service shall establish and maintain a program which increases public awareness of I&R services, their objectives, and their value to the community.

Index